DR. AGISA BEGAY

FOODS LISTS
for
KIDNEY DISEASE

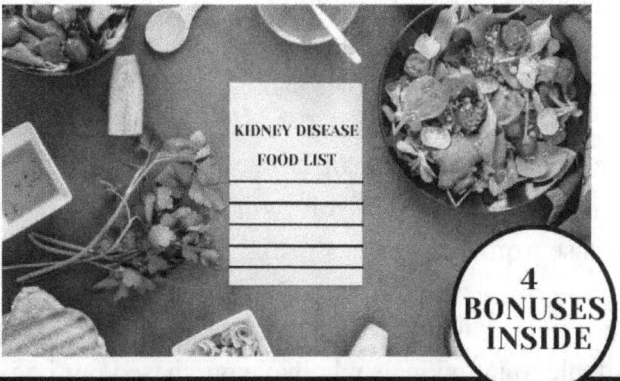

KIDNEY DISEASE
FOOD LIST

4 BONUSES INSIDE

Essential CKD Foods Lists With Low Sodium, Low Potassium, Low Phosphorus Contents + Renal Friendly Recipes and Meal Plans for Chronic Kidney Disease Stage 2, 3, 4 (Diet Guide to Rejuvenate Kidney Health and Avoid Dialysis)

FREE EMAIL CONSULTATION

Dear Reader,

Thank you for choosing to embark on the healing journey with our book. Your support means the world to us, and we are deeply grateful for your trust.

As a token of our appreciation, we would like to offer you a unique opportunity. We are delighted to provide a complimentary email consultation where you can address any questions or challenges you may encounter while implementing the principles shared in our book.

Simply send me an email at medlifeconsults@gmail.com and within 24 hours, you will receive a personalized response from me.

Please note that this free consultation offer is exclusively available to individuals who have purchased our book.

Once again, we extend our heartfelt thanks for your support, and we look forward to assisting you on your healing journey

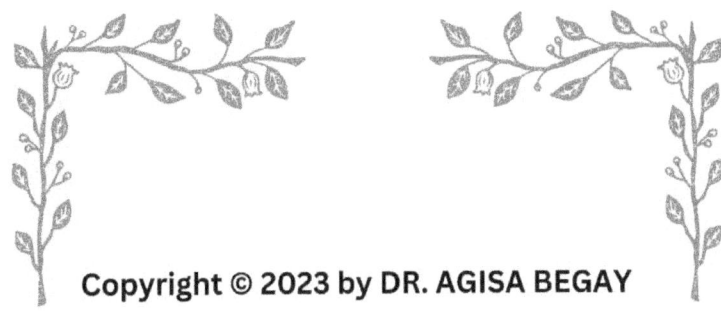

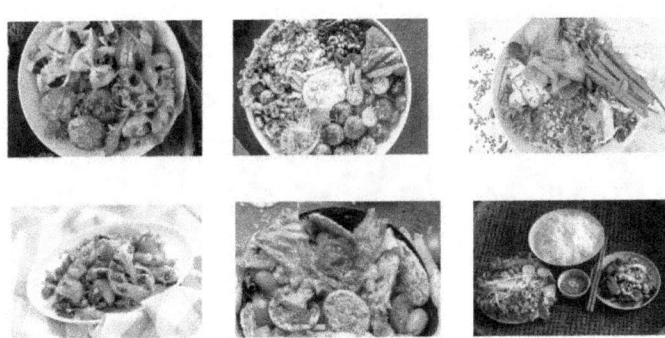

Table of Contents

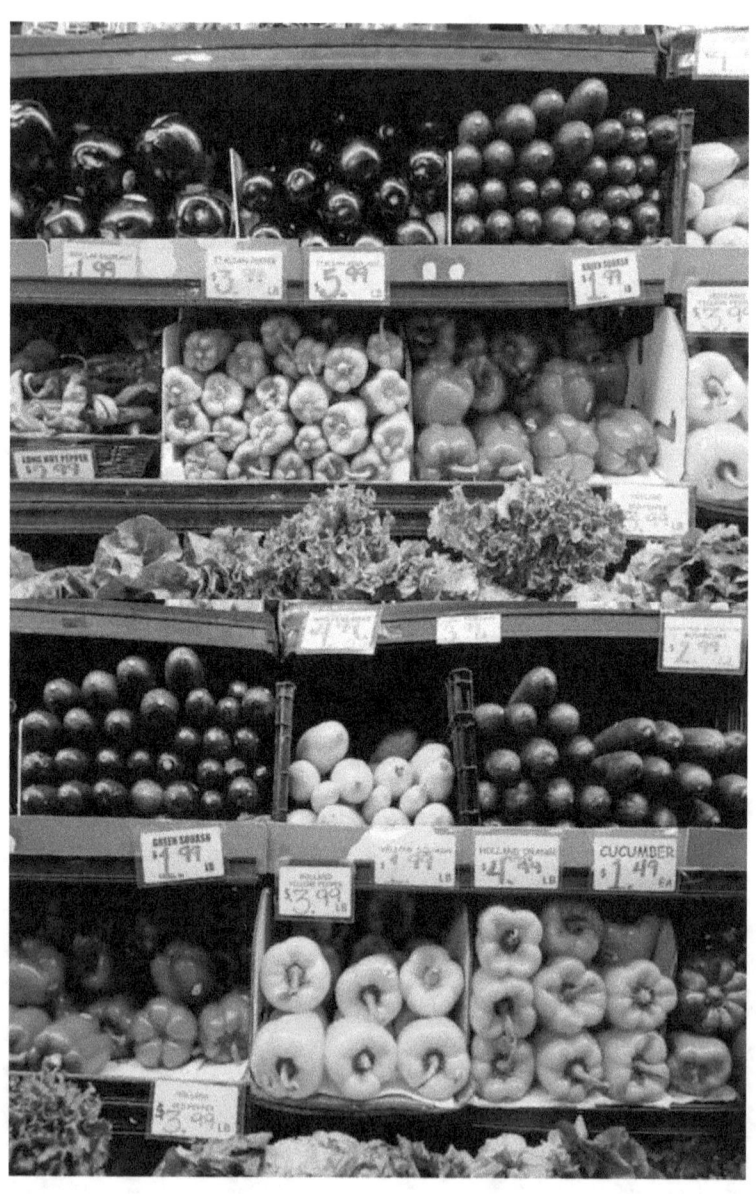

My Experience with Kidney Disease

I grew up with this close friend called Betty Rowlands. We shared almost everything together: the same birth month, the same classroom in school, the same playground at home, and the same church down the street. Betty was the only child, as I was to my parents. We grew up as sisters with separate parents. Betty was blessed to have my parents look out for her like she was theirs. Her family was also nice to me.

Little did I know that fate and the future wouldn't be nice to Betty. Her dad passed away a few days after Betty's 13th birthday in a plane crash, sending her mother, who was undergoing diabetes treatment, into depression, and after some time, high blood pressure set in due to the shock.

Betty's parents have known each other since college and have grown to be one of the best couples I have ever seen. It was natural to see Betty's mom (Mrs. Kate Rowlands) go into depression, but what looks surprising to me is that Mrs. Kate went back to her old life of smoking, drinking, and drugs, just to free up her memories of her husband.

Betty's dad's death was a great loss to the family and to us as friends. But the most concerning situation was the lifestyle Betty's mom was adopting, even with her diabetic and hypertensive state. The smoking, drugs, and alcoholic lifestyle gave her little time to consider her nutritional needs.

Three years after Mr. Rowlands death, it didn't seem like Mrs. Rowlands was ready to give up on the lifestyle she had chosen for herself. It didn't take long before the least expected happened on one calm Saturday evening: Betty's mom was reported to have broken down and was admitted to the nearby health care down the street.

She was examined and diagnosed with stage 3 kidney disease, a condition that erupted from poorly managed diabetes and hypertension.

This news broke Betty as well as myself. Betty's mom was in a very critical state, as she was battling for not only her life but also to get past those memories about her husband.

She was subjected primarily to dieting by her doctor; she was assigned to work closely with a dietician as well as a dieting guide. Her meals and food choices were modeled to meet her body's nutrition needs to help rejuvenate her kidneys and avoid dialysis.

During this period, my family was very helpful to Mrs. Kate Rowlands, as she is a cherished family friend. My mom, who was a seasoned chef, occasionally helped her with some of the dishes, but what actually made the big difference was her personalized food list book recommended by her dietician. Mrs. Kate Rowlands meticulously followed every food tip and savored every recipe as prescribed; she became very mindful and selective with her eating, as she was already seeing the dividends; her blood sugar levels moderated, her blood pressure stabilized, and, to her greatest surprise, her waistline reduced! She has not only cut down on that stubborn belly fat; she has also significantly optimized her kidney function and her energy levels. This was one of the biggest wonders I have ever seen; her doctors, neighbors, and everyone around her marveled at this transformation. The more she used the book, the better she became; her skin and body metabolism were perfect.

These selected foods were what she needed to prevent her kidney disease from progressing. Gradually, Mrs. Kate has turned to a symbol of reference, even to the extent that my mom had to get a copy of this exact food guide. To be frank, the recipes in this guide were exceptional; we savored these delights almost every day. I never imagined this dish would taste this good, to be honest!

I was happy to see the relief in Betty's face after a rough three years since her father's death; at least she was not going to lose her mom anytime soon, as she had thought. Sharing these stories from my childhood memories is a sign of my respect and love for Mrs. Kate Rowlands and Betty, my dear friend.

I am dedicating this book to Mrs. Kate Rowlands, who was resilient in the midst of adversity, giving dieting a chance in her life, and to the countless individuals out there battling with kidney disease.

I never knew that one day I would be sharing these stories of my childhood. I am glad I am doing this right now, and I will be reaching millions of readers through this book.

I know we still have as many Mrs. Rowlands around the world, ready to give the ultimate power of dieting and healthy food choices a chance. My advice to you is to keep on believing that kidney disease isn't a death sentence; it's a hurdle that you will surely cross over. I am ready to give you a shoulder to lean on with this book. Keep reading; **I love you.**

Dear Valued Reader,

Thank you for choosing our cookbook from the sea of options available. Your decision to embrace heart-healthy, plant-based living with us means the world. We invite you to share your thoughts by dropping a polite review on the website. Your feedback fuels our journey, and we're sincerely appreciative. Let your words be the heartbeat of our shared commitment to well-being. We also humbly ask you to consider checking out and following our author central page; with this, you will be exposed to a wealth of other books by this author.

With gratitude,

DR. AGISA BEGAY

Introduction

Welcome, my dear readers, to a journey through the world of kidney health. This guide is meticulously crafted to help you understand and care for your kidneys better. This book goes beyond the renal food list. In these pages of this essential guide, we'll explore what kidneys do, how they get sick, and what we can do to keep them healthy.

In Part 1 of our book, we'll learn about kidneys, their functions, and what happens when they're not well. We'll talk about the signs and symptoms of kidney problems, what causes them, the diagnosis, and what you can do if you're at risk. We'll also explore treatments for kidney disease.

In Part 2 of our book, we will look into managing diabetes, high blood pressure, and kidney health. We'll evaluate how things like diabetes and high blood pressure affect our kidneys. We'll learn about the glycemic index and how eating in accordance with it can help manage your kidneys and diabetic health.

In Part three of our book, readers will be introduced to a world of smarter and healthier food decisions.
We'll dive into food choices that help our kidneys and those that might harm them. We'll talk about avoiding processed foods and reducing inflammation in our bodies by eating better. This will take us to part four of our book, where we will dwell on the potassium, phosphorus, and sodium counters. In this part of our book, we'll provide a list of foods that are good for kidneys, like low-potassium options, recipes, and helpful tips for making healthier meals.

After having the required knowledge of eating with the glycemic index rhythm, making smarter food choices, and eating to balance your electrolytes (potassium, sodium, and phosphorus levels), we will delve into the world of renal-friendly recipes to keep you off your surgeon's door. Here, you will be introduced to a handful of healthy recipes (soups and stew, mains, snacks and appetizers, side dishes, and salads). These dishes constitute essential nutrients capable of optimizing your kidneys, improving kidney function, and avoiding dialysis.

Beyond these chapters, there are bonuses included—like a 30-day meal plan to improve kidney function, information about drugs to avoid with kidney issues, and a weekly meal planner to help you on your journey to better kidney health.

Join us on this exploration of kidney wellness, where each page brings you closer to understanding your kidneys and making choices that keep them strong.

Part 1

Understanding Kidney Disease

What Are Kidneys and How Do They Function?

The kidneys, which are roughly the size of a fist, are located on either side of the spine at the lowest level of the rib cage. Each kidney has up to a million functional units called nephrons. A nephron consists of a filtering unit of tiny blood vessels known as a glomerulus attached to a tubule. Blood is filtered as it enters the glomerulus, and the leftover fluid passes down the tubule.

Chemicals and water are added to or removed from this filtered fluid in the tubule according on the demands of the body, with the end product being the urine we expel.

Every 24 hours, the kidneys execute their life-sustaining function of filtering and returning around 200 quarts of fluid to the bloodstream. Roughly two quarts of urine are evacuated from the body, and roughly 198 quarts are retrieved. The urine we expel has been kept in our bladder for 1 to 8 hours.

What Is the Role of the Kidneys?

Most individuals are aware that one of the kidneys' primary functions is to eliminate waste materials and excess fluid from the body. The urine removes these waste materials and extra fluid. Urine production comprises highly complex excretion and re-absorption steps. This mechanism is expected to keep the body's chemical equilibrium steady and going.

The kidneys are responsible for the vital regulation of the body's salt, potassium, and acid content. In addition, the kidneys create hormones that influence the operation of other organs. A hormone produced by the kidneys, for example, increases red blood cell formation. Other hormones produced by the kidneys aid in blood pressure regulation and calcium metabolism.

The kidneys are designed to carry out the following tasks:

- Eliminate waste from the body
- Drug removal from the body
- Fluid equilibrium in the body
- Releases hormones that modulate blood pressure
- Produces a form of vitamin D that is active and promotes strong, healthy bones
- Regulate red blood cell production

The kidneys will continue to function in its proper and healthy state until it is altered by certain factors, capable of infecting it and thus bringing it to a *"disease"* state. This brings us to the term **Chronic Kidney Disease**.

What Exactly Is Chronic Kidney Disease and What Causes It?

Chronic kidney disease is characterized as having some type of renal anomaly, or "marker," such as protein in the urine for three months or more and having impaired kidney function.

Chronic renal disease can be caused by a variety of factors. Diabetes and high blood pressure are two disorders that can harm the kidneys. Some kidney diseases are hereditary (run in families).

Others are congenital, meaning that people are given birth to with a defect that affects their kidneys. Some of the most prevalent forms and causes of kidney injury are as follows.

Diabetes is a condition in which your body does not produce enough insulin or cannot properly use normal levels of insulin. This causes a spike in blood sugar, which can cause problems in many sections of your body. Diabetes is the most common cause of renal disease.

Another prominent cause of kidney disease and concomitant consequences such as heart attacks and strokes is high blood pressure (also known as hypertension). This occurs when the force of blood against your artery walls increases, causing you to have high blood pressure. Controlling hypertension lowers the risk of consequences such as chronic renal disease.

Glomerulonephritis is a condition that involves inflammation of the glomeruli, which are small filtering units in the kidney. Glomerulonephritis can occur unexpectedly, such as after strep throat, and the individual may recover. However, the condition can advance slowly over time, causing increasing loss of kidney function.

The most prevalent inherited kidney illness is polycystic kidney disease. It is distinguished by the creation of kidney cysts, which increase over time and can result in major kidney damage and even renal failure. Other inherited kidney illnesses include Alport's Syndrome, primary hyperoxaluria, and cystinuria.

Kidney stones are fairly common, and they can cause considerable discomfort in your back and side as they pass. Kidney stones can be caused by a variety of factors, including a hereditary disease that causes excessive calcium absorption from diets and urinary tract infections or blockages. Medication and diet can sometimes assist to avoid recurring stone development. When stones are too large to travel through the body, procedures may be performed to remove the stones or break them down into small fragments that can pass through the body.

Urinary tract infections arise when germs enter the urinary tract, causing symptoms such as pain and/or burning during urination, as well as an increased need to urinate. These infections most commonly attack the bladder, but they can also extend to the kidneys and cause fever and back pain.

Kidneys can also be affected by congenital disorders. These typically entail an issue in the urinary tract while a kid is developing in its mother's womb. One of the most common occurs when a valve-like mechanism between the bladder and the ureter (urine tube) fails to function properly, allowing urine to back up (reflux) into the kidneys, causing infections and perhaps kidney damage.

Toxins and drugs can also cause renal issues. Long-term use of a significant number of over-the-counter pain medications may cause kidney damage. Other pharmaceuticals, pollutants, insecticides, and *"street"* drugs like heroin and crack can also harm the kidneys.

What Are the Symptoms of Kidney Disease?

In most cases, kidney disease affects both kidneys. Wastes and extra fluid may accumulate in the body if the kidneys' ability to filter blood is severely impaired by disease. Although many forms of kidney disease may not develop symptoms until late in the disease's progression, there are six kidney disease warning signs, which are as follows:

- Blood pressure that is too high.
- Urine containing blood and/or protein.
- A creatinine and blood urea nitrogen (BUN) level that is higher than usual. BUN and creatinine are waste products that accumulate in your blood when your kidney function is compromised.

- GFR (glomerular filtration rate) less than 60. GFR measures renal function.
- Urinating becomes more frequent, especially at night; urinating becomes difficult or unpleasant.
- Puffiness around the eyes, as well as swelling in the hands and feet.

Immediately you observe any of these, you are required to head straight to your doctor for diagnosis. As you read on, we will delve into diagnosis and everything you need to know.

How Does Chronic Kidney Disease Get Diagnosed?

The key to preventing kidney disease from advancing to kidney failure is early detection and treatment of chronic renal disease. To diagnose early kidney disease, few simple tests can be performed. They are as follows:

A protein test for the urine. The albumin to creatinine ratio (ACR) calculates the amount of albumin in your urine. A high level of protein in your urine could indicate that your kidney's filtration units have been harmed by illness. Because one good result could be related to a fever or strenuous exercise, your doctor will want to confirm your test over a period of many weeks. A blood creatinine test. Your doctor should compute your glomerular filtration rate (GFR) based on your results, as well as your age, race, gender, and other characteristics. Your GFR indicates how well your kidneys work.

These tests are especially critical for patients who are at a higher risk of developing chronic renal disease.

If you fall into one of these categories or believe you may be at elevated risk for kidney disease, speak with your doctor about getting tested.

Risk Factors for Chronic Kidney Disease

In most cases, CKD are caused by disorders that put a burden on your kidneys. It is frequently the result of several separate circumstances interacting to generate issues. CKD can potentially exacerbate the underlying diseases. The two most significant risk factors are:

1. **Diabetes:** Having too much sugar (glucose) in your blood can harm your kidneys over time, leading to complications that can trigger kidney disease.

2. **High blood pressure:** High blood pressure puts strain on the small blood arteries in your kidneys, affecting how they function. Other conditions can also provide a risk for CKD, these conditions include:

3. **Cardiovascular illness:** commonly known as heart disease, refers to a variety of conditions

that affect your heart and blood arteries and can put strain on your kidneys. Examples of coronary illness are:

- *Coronary artery disease* which indicates that your arteries have grown clogged.

- *A heart attack* (a clot that prevents blood from flowing to your heart)

- *Heart failure* (Having issues with your heart muscle, valve, or heart beat)

4. **Kidney infections**: This occur when bacteria from your bladder enter one or both of your kidneys. If you have a lot of kidney infections over a long period of time and don't treat them, they can cause irreversible damage, though this is unlikely.

5. **Long-term consistent usage of certain medications:** primarily pain relievers such as ibuprofen, aspirin, and naproxen. Occasional use is not an issue. However, if you take them every day for an extended period of time, they may affect your kidneys, particularly pain relievers that combine two or more medications with caffeine or codeine.

6. **Autoimmune disorders:** This occurs when immune system incorrectly targets your body, can cause inflammation and damage to the kidney filters.

7. **Age:** Those over 60 years old are at higher risk, and one in every five people over 60 in the UK has some form of renal disease, according to some data.

8. **Hereditary:** People who have a history of renal illness in their family stands at risk of developing kidney disease.

9. **Race:** Individuals from an African American, Hispanic American, Asian or Pacific Islander, or American Indian, African or South Asian descent have the probability of having kidney disease.

What Should You Do If You at Risk of CKD

If you are concerned about your risk of CKD, the best thing to do is to consult with your doctor.

It can be frightening to discuss with your doctor whether you are at danger of a major health problem, but it is critical that you do so if you are concerned. Your doctor can: run tests to assess your kidney health; they may reveal no problems and put your mind at ease.

Look for underlying conditions associated with CKD. To lessen the likelihood of current conditions contributing to CKD, ensure sure they are effectively controlled.

Is It Possible To Successfully Treat Kidney Disease?

Many renal problems can be successfully addressed with the right knowledge and approach. Controlling disorders such as diabetes and high blood pressure can help prevent or slow the progression of kidney disease. Kidney stones and urinary tract infections are frequently treatable. Chronic renal disease can sometimes progress to kidney failure, necessitating dialysis or kidney transplantation. Treating high blood pressure with angiotensin converting enzyme (ACE) inhibitors, as well as following a renal-friendly diet, can sometimes assist to halt the progression of chronic kidney disease. The healthy eating approach has grown in importance in the fight against CKD throughout the years. Much research is being conducted in order to develop more effective treatments for all illnesses that can cause chronic kidney disease.

What is the Treatment for Kidney Failure?

Hemodialysis, peritoneal dialysis, or kidney transplantation can all be used to treat renal failure. Hemodialysis (artificial kidney) treatment can be done at a dialysis unit or at home. Hemodialysis is typically conducted three times each week. Peritoneal dialysis is often performed at home on a daily basis. Continuous Ambulatory Peritoneal Dialysis does not require the use of a machine, whereas Continuous Cycling Peritoneal Dialysis does. A kidney expert can explain the various options and assist individuals in making the best treatment decisions for themselves and their families.

Our book will focus on the dietary approach in managing and preventing kidney disease and dialysis. Certain food possess healing components far beyond what you can imagine. In the chapters ahead, We will delve into making these recipes.

Kidney transplants are extremely successful. The kidney could come from a deceased donor or a living donor, who could be a relative, friend, or even a stranger who donates a kidney to anyone in need of a transplant.

I hope you are enjoying your time with our book, kindly contact me for consultations if need be @ medlifeconsults@gmail.com. As a token of appreciation, I humbly request you consider dropping a polite review in the website about my book. This kind gesture of yours means the world to me as an independent publisher, thank you and do have a wonderful time with the contents ahead.

PART 2

Managing Diabetes, High Blood Pressure, and Kidney Health

Diabetes and high blood pressure are commonly referred to as *"silent killers,"* because many people are unaware that they have these conditions and hence do not seek treatment. Chronic kidney disease (CKD) can develop from uncontrolled diabetes and/or uncontrolled high blood pressure.

Here are some facts to consider:

- Diabetes is the leading cause of kidney disease in the United States, affecting 6% of the population.

- High blood pressure affects one in every four Americans and is the second largest cause of renal disease.

- Anyone who has diabetes, high blood pressure, or a family history of these disorders is predisposed to kidney disease.

- Kidney disease affects 20 million Americans, or one in every ten persons.

- Another 20 million Americans are at risk of kidney disease but are unaware of it.

- African Americans, Latinos, Hispanics, Pacific Islanders, Native Americans, and seniors (those 65 and older) are more likely to acquire renal disease.

Another leading causes of kidney disease and kidney failure is high blood pressure (hypertension). When blood pressure is high, there is a lot of stress inside the blood vessels, which can cause harm. These blood vessels can constrict **("close off")**, resulting in a heart attack, stroke, or renal failure.

High glucose and cholesterol levels can potentially harm blood vessels. As a result, those with diabetes who simultaneously have hypertension are at an increased risk of blood vessel damage. It normally takes years for blood vessels to totally constrict, and blood vessel damage can be slowed or reversed with treatment.

High blood pressure can only be diagnosed by having your blood pressure taken by someone who is trained in taking blood pressures. In most cases, there are no evident symptoms of high blood pressure. If you have diabetes, blood pressure that is more than 130/80 is considered high.

Blood pressure should be monitored several times during the day because it might change throughout the day and it is common to have readings higher than 130/80 on occasion. Blood pressure often rises in the middle of the day and falls at night while you sleep. If feasible, take your blood pressure from your left arm, and do it after you've rested for 5-10 minutes. Your left arm should be relaxed at heart level.

As part of your blood pressure management, your healthcare providers may ask you to check your blood pressure at home and record the numbers.

There are numerous methods for controlling your blood pressure. The first stage is to alter one's lifestyle.
Blood pressure can be affected directly by your diet and lifestyle. Too much sodium (salt), alcohol, or coffee, for example, may raise your blood pressure. Your weight has an impact on your blood pressure as well. Weight gain causes fluid retention, and the excess fat releases

hormones that can raise blood pressure. Excess weight makes the heart work harder. Exercise on a regular basis can help you lose weight faster.

Exercise can reduce your systolic blood pressure (the highest number in a blood pressure reading) by 4 to 9 mm of mercury on average. Exercise can even help some people minimize their need for blood pressure medication. Regular exercise also strengthens your heart, allowing it to pump more blood with less effort. Even if you don't have high blood pressure, regular exercise can help keep it down as you become older. Weight loss, lowering sodium, alcohol, and caffeine in your diet, reducing stress, and boosting exercise are all significant components of blood pressure regulation.

What Is the Glycemic Index and How Can It Help My Kidney Health?

The glycemic index is a scale that determines how much a food affects blood sugar levels. A food's glycemic index is affected by several factors, including ripeness, nutrient makeup, and cooking method.

The glycemic index is a tool that is frequently used to encourage better blood sugar control.

The glycemic index of a food is influenced by several factors, including its nutrient composition, cooking method, ripeness, and amount of processing.

The glycemic index can help you lose weight, lower your blood sugar levels, and lower your cholesterol by encouraging you to be more conscious of what you put on your plate.

This section of the book delves deeper into the glycemic index, explaining what it is, how it might effect your health, and how to apply it.

What exactly is the glycemic index?

The glycemic index (GI) of foods determines how much they raise blood sugar levels. Foods are categorized as low, medium, or high glycemic on a scale of 0-100.

The lower a food's GI, the less it may affect your blood sugar levels.

The three GI ratings are as follows:

- Low: 55 or lower
- Medium (56-69)
- High: 70 or higher

Those high in refined carbs and sugar digest faster and have a higher GI, whereas those high in protein, fat, or fiber have a lower GI. Foods with no GI include meat, fish, poultry, nuts, seeds, herbs, spices, and oils.

Other factors influencing a food's GI include its ripeness, cooking style, the type of sugar it contains, and the amount of processing it has experienced.

Keep in mind that the glycemic index (GI) is not the same as the glycemic load (GL). Unlike the GI, which does not include the quantity of food consumed, the GL considers the number of carbs in a portion of a food to evaluate how it may alter blood sugar levels. As a result, it's vital to consider both the glycemic index and the glycemic load when selecting meals to help promote appropriate blood sugar levels. Below are some reasons why taking a Low GI food is of importance to your health.

Benefits:

A low glycemic diet may provide a number of health benefits, including:

- **Improved blood sugar control:** Numerous studies have demonstrated that a low GI diet lowers blood sugar levels and improves blood sugar management in people with type 2 diabetes.

- **Weight loss:** According to certain studies, following a low GI diet may boost short-term weight loss. More research is needed to assess its impact on long-term weight management.

- **Benefits People with fatty liver:** A low-glycemic diet could help reduce liver fat and liver enzyme levels in patients with non-alcoholic fatty liver disease.

How to Follow a Low Glycemic Index Diet

A healthy, low glycemic diet should consist primarily of low GI foods such as:

- **Fruits:** apples, berries, oranges, lemons, limes, grapefruit

- **Non-starchy vegetables:** broccoli, cauliflower, carrots, spinach, tomatoes

- **Whole grains:** quinoa, barley, buckwheat, farro, oats

- **Legumes:** lentils, black beans, chickpeas, kidney beans

Foods without a GI value or with a very low GI can also be enjoyed as part of a balanced low glycemic diet. They include:

- **Meat:** beef, bison, lamb, pork

- **Seafood:** tuna, salmon, shrimp, mackerel, anchovies, sardines

- **Poultry:** chicken, turkey, duck, goose

- **Oils:** olive oil, coconut oil, avocado oil, vegetable oil

- **Nuts:** almonds, macadamia nuts, walnuts, pistachios

- **Seeds:** chia seeds, sesame seeds, hemp seeds, flax seeds

- **Herbs and spices:** turmeric, black pepper, cumin, dill, basil, rosemary, cinnamon

- **Some pastas:** Semolina and whole grain pasta

Foods with a high GI include:

- **Bread:** white bread, bagels, naan, pita bread

- **Rice:** white rice, jasmine rice, arborio rice

- **Cereals:** instant oats, breakfast cereals

- **Starchy vegetables:** mashed potatoes, potatoes, french fries

- **Baked goods:** cake, doughnuts, cookies, croissants, muffins

- **Snacks:** chocolate, crackers, microwave popcorn, chips, pretzels

- **Sugar-sweetened beverages:** soda, fruit juice, sports drinks

Ideally, you should try to replace these high GI foods with foods that have a lower GI whenever possible.

Glycemic index of foods

Knowing the GI of regularly consumed goods can be useful if you follow a low glycemic diet. The GI values of a few substances are listed below.

Fruits

- Apples: 36
- Strawberries: 41
- Dates: 42
- Oranges: 43
- Banana: 51
- Mango: 51
- Blueberries: 53
- Pineapple: 59
- Watermelon: 76

Vegetables

- Carrots (boiled): 39
- Plantains (boiled): 66

- Sweet potatoes (boiled): 63
- Pumpkin (boiled): 74
- Potatoes (boiled): 78

Grains

- Barley: 28
- Quinoa: 53
- Rolled oats: 55
- Couscous: 65
- Popcorn: 65
- Brown rice: 68
- White rice: 73
- Whole wheat bread: 74
- White bread: 75

Legumes

- Soybeans: 16
- Kidney beans: 24
- Chickpeas: 28
- Lentils: 32

Dairy products and dairy alternatives

- Soymilk: 34
- Skim milk: 37
- Whole milk: 39
- Ice cream: 51
- Rice milk: 86

Sweeteners

- Fructose: 15
- Coconut sugar: 54
- Maple syrup: 54
- Honey: 61
- Table sugar: 65

Cooking and ripening effects on Glycemic Index

The cooking process used for various foods can influence the glycemic index.

Fried foods, for example, have a high fat content, which can impede sugar absorption in the circulation and lower the GI.

Meanwhile, roasting and baking can break down resistant starch, a type of starch that resists digestion and is present in foods such as beans, potatoes, and oats, raising the GI.

When compared to other cooking processes, boiling is expected to help retain more of the resistant starch and result in a lower GI.

The longer you cook foods like pasta or rice, the more digestible the starch content becomes, and hence the higher the GI. As a result, it's advisable to only cook these meals until they're al dente, which means they're still firm when biting into them.

In addition to the cooking method, the degree of ripeness of some fruits, such as bananas, may impact their GI. This is due to the fact that the amount of resistant starch reduces during the ripening process, resulting in a higher GI. For example, fully matured bananas have a GI of 51, but under-ripe bananas have a GI of 30.

Glycemic Index and Diabetes Nutrition

Eating according to the GI can help you better regulate your blood sugar levels after meals. The GI can also assist you in determining appropriate food pairings.

Eating multiple low GI fruits and vegetables in conjunction with a high GI food, for example, will help you maintain better blood sugar control. Other ideas include combining beans with rice, nut butter with toast, and tomato sauce with spaghetti.

Utilizing the glycemic index for diabetic health

Choosing foods with a low glycemic index can help you maintain a healthy blood sugar level. However, you must strictly adhere to the prescribed serving sizes. Glycemic indexes aren't just for diabetics.

Those attempting to lose weight or reduce hunger use the GI as a diet since it can limit appetite. Because food takes longer to digest in the body, a person can feel fuller for a longer period of time.

The glycemic index (GI) is a dietary metric that can help you rate the quality of carbohydrates you consume.

The glycemic index evaluates how quickly carbohydrates in a particular food affect your blood sugar levels.

Foods are classified as low, medium, or high on the glycemic index based on how quickly they elevate blood sugar levels when compared to glucose or white bread (both of which have a glycemic index rating of 100).

You can reduce blood sugar spikes by eating meals with a low glycemic index.

Furthermore, eating foods with a high glycemic index will cause your blood sugar to rise dramatically. It may also result in a greater post-meal blood sugar level.

A food's glycemic index can be affected by a variety of things. These considerations include the food's composition and cooking method. When foods are combined together, their glycemic index changes.

The glycemic index of a food is not based on a typical serving of that item. Carrots, for example, have a high glycemic index, but you'd have to consume a pound and a half to achieve the quantity measured for carrot glycemic index.

An alternative metric, known as glycemic load, comes to the picture when ever glycemic index is mentioned; this metric considers both the rate of digestion and the amount present in a typical portion of a food. This may be a more accurate technique of determining the effect of a carbohydrate food on blood sugar levels.

When assigning a glycemic rating to a food, several elements are considered.

These elements are as follows:

- **Acidity:** Highly acidic foods, such as pickles, have a lower GI than meals that are not. This explains why lactic acid-based breads, such as sourdough bread, have a lower GI than white bread.

- **Time to cook:** The longer an item is cooked, the higher its GI rating. When you cook something, the starch or carbohydrates begin to break down.

- **Fiber Content:** Fiber-rich foods have lower glycemic indexes in general. Because of the fibrous coatings on beans and seeds, the body breaks them down more slowly. As a result, they are lower on the glycemic index than foods without this coating.

- **Processing:** In general, the more processed a food is, the higher it ranks on the glycemic index. Fruit juice, for example, has a higher GI rating than fresh fruits.

- **Ripeness:** The higher the GI of a fruit or vegetable, the riper it is.

While each rule has exceptions, here are some general rules to consider when evaluating the possible blood sugar impact of a certain dish.

PART 3

Making Smarter and Healthier Food Decisions

In the part three of our book, we will delve into making not only smart food choices, but healthier food decision capable of giving us an edge over dialysis.

What Foods Aid in Kidney Repair?

Because sick kidneys cannot remove waste items from the body as well as healthy kidneys, it is critical to watch food and hydration intake if you have chronic renal disease. Here are the top kidney-friendly foods to help you repair your kidneys and live a healthier life:

- **Apples:** Apples are rich in pectin, a type of soluble fiber. It possesses the ability to decrease cholesterol and glucose levels. It has a lot of antioxidants. Fresh apples are also rich in vitamin C.
- **Blueberries:** Blueberries are a high-fiber, low-calorie source of vitamin C. According to research, it has the ability to protect against cancer and heart disease, as well as providing benefits to brain health.

- **Fish:** Omega-3 fatty acids are abundant in salmon, mackerel, tuna, herring, and sardines. It is required for blood clotting and the formation of cell membranes in the brain. According to scientific research, it may reduce the chance of an irregular heartbeat, cut triglyceride levels, and slightly lower blood pressure. They may be useful in illnesses such as cancer, autoimmune disease, and inflammatory bowel disease.

- **Kale:** Kale is high in vitamins A and C, calcium, and a variety of minerals. It also contains carotenoids and flavonoids, which are good for eye health and cancer prevention. It also contains vitamin K, a naturally occurring blood thinner. It has a considerable amount of potassium. As a result, dialysis patients must try to avoid it.

- **Spinach:** Spinach is abundant in vitamins A, C, and K, as well as folate. Spinach contains beta-carotene, which helps to increase your immunity and protect your vision. It also contains a lot of magnesium.

- **Sweet potato:** Sweet potato has a low sugar content and a high soluble fiber content. This makes you feel fuller.

Other healthful foods that can help prevent kidney disease include:

- Cranberries
- Arugula
- Raspberries
- Strawberries
- Plums
- Pineapples
- Peaches
- Cabbage
- Cauliflower
- Asparagus
- Beans
- Celery
- Cucumber
- Onions
- Bell peppers
- Radishes
- Summer squash
- Garlic
- Egg whites without yolks
- Shiitake mushrooms

- Water

- Olive oil

- Skinless chicken has less potassium and sodium than the skin on

- Macadamia nuts

- Turnips are a great alternative to potatoes and winter squash

What effect does a kidney-friendly diet have?

A renal-friendly diet will help in the prevention of additional kidney damage. Some foods and fluids must be restricted so that other fluids and minerals, such as electrolytes, do not accumulate in your body. You must also ensure that you are obtaining enough protein, calories, vitamins, and minerals in your everyday diet. There are a few foods you should avoid if you have early-stage renal disease. However, as your sickness progresses, you must be more mindful of your regular food consumption.

What foods should I avoid if I have renal disease?

Many foods that are part of a regular healthy diet may not be suitable for you if you have renal disease.

If you have renal illness, your doctor may advise you to limit specific foods, such as:

- **Avoid using table salt and high-sodium seasonings:** Sodium influences your blood pressure and aids in the maintenance of your body's water level. Salt should be avoided if you have ankle edema, high blood pressure, difficulty breathing, or fluid buildup around your heart and lungs. You should limit your daily salt intake to fewer than 1,500 mg. Instead of salt, use spices or herbs. Avoid packaged foods and check labels when buying. Concentrate on fresh, home-cooked meals. Within a week or two, you will become accustomed to eating foods with little or no salt.

- **Potassium:** When you have kidney illness, elevated potassium levels in your blood can cause major heart difficulties. This mineral keeps your neurons and muscles in good operating order. Potassium-rich foods include tomatoes, oranges, bananas, potatoes, avocados, broccoli, and whole-grain bread. Consume salads, apples, and carrots. To assist your body get rid of excess potassium, your doctor may recommend a potassium binder. Apples, cranberries, strawberries, cabbage, cauliflower, and cucumber may be recommended by the doctor.

- **Protein:** While protein is necessary for your body, eating too much of it causes your kidneys to work harder and may worsen renal disease. Consult your dietician to establish the best protein combination and amount for you. Foods like meat, seafood, and dairy items may need to be cut.

- **Phosphorus:** Phosphorus is a mineral that helps to maintain your bones strong and healthy. In renal disease, your kidneys are unable to remove excess phosphorus from your blood. It may cause bone deterioration and further harm to your blood vessels, eyes, and heart. You could potentially develop heart disease. Avoid foods high in phosphorus, such as meat, fish, dairy, beans, nuts, whole-grain bread, packaged foods, and dark-colored drinks. If you have advanced kidney disease, your doctor may urge you to limit your daily intake of phosphorus-rich foods to less than 1000 mg. Choose low-phosphorus foods such fresh fruits and vegetables, corn, rice, and cereal.

- **Calcium:** Your doctor may also urge you to avoid taking over-the-counter calcium supplements and to limit your intake of calcium-rich foods like dairy products. Foods high in calcium tend to be high in phosphorus as well.

- **Fluids:** In general, you should keep your body's water level stable. However, if you have early-stage renal disease, you should minimize your fluid intake. Because damaged kidneys cannot eliminate excess fluid, drinking too much fluid can be hazardous to your health. It can potentially cause hypertension, edema, and heart failure. It can also cause excess fluid to accumulate around your lungs, making breathing harder.

You should also limit your intake of foods high in water, such as ice cream, gelatin, watermelon, and grapes.

Your doctor will advise you to reduce the potassium, phosphorus, and protein levels in your diet depending on the stage of your renal illness.

What fruit is harmful to the kidneys?

Although fruits are generally healthy to the diet, the following fruits are high in potassium and should be avoided by individuals with renal disease:

- Bananas
- Avocados
- Oranges and grapefruit juice (citrus fruits and drinks).
- Prunes and their juice
- Apricots
- Dates and raisins are examples of dried fruits.
- Melons like honeydew and cantaloupe

In patients with kidney disease, the citric acid in oranges may increase the chance of developing kidney stones. Salt and salt substitutes containing potassium should be avoided. If the patient's potassium or other harmful substance levels rise, he or she may need dialysis.

Ultra-Processed Foods and Kidney Disease; Is There a Link?

A journey down any aisle of a grocery or convenience shop will reveal a plethora of quick and easy-to-make ultra-processed foods and beverages. They're excellent, and you can eat them right away or after a few minutes in the microwave or on the stove.

Isn't it too good to be true? According to a recently published study, it most likely is.

The relationship between highly processed meals and renal disease

Over a 24-year period, a research study monitored over 14,000 persons without kidney illness to investigate if ultra-processed foods (UPFs) increased the chance of acquiring kidney disease.

The results may surprise you.

Those who ingested high levels of UPFs had a 24% increased risk of getting renal disease: over 5000 participants in the UPF-rich diet group got chronic kidney disease.

It's becoming evident that food is medicine: the appropriate diet can help avoid kidney illness, but other foods, especially when consumed in big amounts, can actually induce renal disease." NKF Chief Scientific Officer Kerry Willis, Ph.D. said. "In this study, there was a direct correlation between the amount of UPF consumed and the risk of CKD," said the researchers, "which should concern everyone: doctors, patients, parents, and public health officials."

What Exactly Are Ultra-Processed Foods?

They are highly processed foods that are high in artificial additives, sugar, refined carbohydrates, saturated and trans fats, and sodium. They don't have a lot of fiber, protein, or minerals. Furthermore, the packaging or packaging process may contaminate the product.

Foods that have been ultra-processed include:

- soda or carbonated soft drinks
- packed sugary, fatty, or salty snacks
- cakes, cookies, and sweets
- bundled bread margarine cereals that are mass-produced

- Instant pot Soups and noodles

- cheese and processed meat

Sugar-sweetened beverages and ultra-processed meats were the most dangerous UPFs evaluated, raising the risk of renal disease by 22% and 18%, respectively.

How to Stay Away from Ultra-Processed Foods

In a world that bombards us with commercials and tempts us at every turn, how do we resist ultra-processed foods?

According to the study, replacing even one serving of ultra-processed foods per day with less processed foods reduces the chance of getting renal disease by 6%. Begin with substituting water, fruits, vegetables, almonds, or whole grains for one or two USFs every day.

Here are a few ideas to get you started on your swap:

I'm craving... Soda
Try: Fresh fruit in water, kombucha

I'm craving....Salty packaged snacks like chips
Try: Raw vegetables, homemade sweet potato chips

I'm craving Sweet and salty
Try: Homemade trail mix with low or no-sodium nuts and dried fruit

I'm craving Mass-produced packaged bread
Try: A slice of homemade or bakery-fresh whole wheat bread

I'm craving...Cereals
Try: Overnight steel-cut oats, rolled oats

I'm craving.... Processed meat

Try: Home-cooked carved chicken or turkey breast, boiled eggs

Remember that while these adjustments are healthier, moderation and a varied diet are still essential for living a healthy life. If you have certain dietary requirements or restrictions, a licensed kidney dietitian can assist you in developing a customized plan.

Cost-cutting suggestions to help you avoid processed meals

To get rid of processed goods in your pantry, you may have to be inventive. We're here to assist you. Here are five inexpensive strategies to incorporate more whole foods into your diet without breaking the bank.

- **Visit or start a community garden:** If you don't have enough space to start your own garden, check for a nearby community garden. As you cultivate your own food, you'll have the opportunity to meet new people. If there isn't one nearby, you can help your community by starting your own.

- **Change up your pantry staples:** Dried lentils, beans, and brown rice frequently supply more food and are less expensive than prepared lentils, beans, and brown rice because they take longer to cook. Stock up on these ingredients and prepare them according to the package directions. Some may require overnight soak, but the extra time is well worth it! You can also regulate how much salt goes into the meal, allowing you to consume less sodium.

- **Make a food scrap garden:** Rather than tossing away leftover fruit and vegetable scraps, use them to produce a completely new plant! You can renew fruit from seeds or vegetables from cuttings, for example.

- **Visit farmer's markets:** Farmer's markets are festive places where you may have fun while buying fresh, affordable goods. Because these markets are so active, bring along friends, family, or neighbors. Use this to your advantage by planning excursions and carpooling to save money on gas.

- **Go Frozen:** Fruits and vegetables are frozen at their height of freshness to help preserve nutrients. They last longer and are less expensive than fresh alternatives. Look for frozen fruits and veggies, but be wary of any sauces or combinations that may contain UPFs.

Foods to Avoid That Causes Inflammation

Inflammation is your body's natural defence against substances that are harmful to your health, such as germs, viruses, and poisons.

However, your immune system is complex, and its components might be triggered by unexpected factors, such as particular foods.

Our diets play a considerably larger part in what happens within our bodies than most people believe.

We've all seen the obvious result of continually eating bad foods: **weight gain**. What you may not know is that being overweight is associated with higher levels of inflammation in the body.

The tale of how our dietary habits can cause inflammation does not end there.

An imbalanced diet includes consuming a lot of processed foods, which contain substances that might directly stimulate inflammatory processes. This is less obvious than weight gain.

What foods contribute to inflammation?

The five categories of foods that promote inflammation are as follows:

- Red meat as well as processed meats such as bacon, hot dogs, lunch meats, and cured foods
- White bread, white rice, pasta, and breakfast cereals are some examples of refined grains.
- Snacks such as chips, cookies, crackers, and pastries
- Sodas and other sugary beverages
- Foods that have been fried

These foods have one thing in common: they all have added sugars, saturated fats, and/or trans fats. With the exception of red meat, all of these are processed foods.

Inflammation can also be caused by alcohol.

Furthermore, alcohol is frequently paired with the aforementioned inflammatory foods. Alcoholic drinks become a double whammy when paired with processed carbohydrates, added sweets, or mixed with soda.

Why are these foods inflammatory?

The cells in your body absorb and react differently to processed foods than they do to natural foods.

Your body is designed to metabolize and utilize the nutrients, vitamins, and minerals found in vegetables, fruits, and whole grains. In reality, it requires these things because they assist coordinate vital functions required for survival.

The refined carbohydrates, fats, and grains found in processed foods are a different story. They aren't required. Furthermore, your body doesn't always know what to do with them, especially if you consume a lot of them.

Foods heavy in fat, sugar, and other refined carbohydrates are fundamentally poisonous to our bodies, triggering inflammatory pathways in a variety of direct and indirect ways.

For example, refined vegetable oils added to processed foods can skew your omega-6 to omega-3 fat ratio. Red meat, while not a source of refined fat, can be, because it contains significant levels of omega 6 fats.

Omega-6 and omega-3 fatty acids are essential fatty acids that the body cannot make but that are required for survival. Although foods with a higher omega-6 fatty acid content are typically healthful, consuming a higher proportion of omega-3 fatty acids leads to an increase in inflammatory illnesses overall.

Experts believe that the ideal omega-6 to omega-3 fatty acid ratio is around 2:1, which can help avoid cardiovascular disease and cancer; a 5:1 ratio has also been demonstrated to help prevent various ailments, compared to the 10:1 ratio found in the usual American diet. I propose boosting your omega-3 intake while limiting your omega-6 intake.

This omega-6/omega-3 imbalance activates proinflammatory substances known as cytokines, which contribute to fatty buildup in the arteries, resulting in a persistent inflammatory state (atherosclerosis) and oxidative stress.

In another pathway, here's the way added sugar and refined carbohydrates, both of which are abundant in many processed foods, promote blood sugar increases.

Elevated blood sugar levels activate proinflammatory pathways, and "consistent blood sugar spikes can eventually result to insulin resistance and diabetes, both of which are linked to inflammation."

A diet that promotes processed foods above natural foods is imbalanced and hypercaloric, resulting in weight gain.

As we gain weight, the number of fat cells grows, these cells emit a variety of hormones and chemicals, some of which cause the body to become inflammatory.

The Bottom line is that, these meals can directly activate pro-inflammatory chemicals while also indirectly promoting weight gain, all of which contribute to inflammation in the body.

But... how horrible is it all really?

Most people are unaware of the subtle indicators of eating inflammatory foods.

However, the underlying, chronic inflammation eventually causes symptoms ranging from unpleasant to quite debilitating, such as:

- Chronic fatigue
- Infections that occur on a regular or recurring basis
- Muscle and joint pain
- Insomnia
- Acid reflux, constipation, and diarrhea (all examples of gastrointestinal ailments)
- Depression and anxiety

Another difficulty with being in a pro-inflammatory condition is that it causes oxidative stress, which occurs when harmful waste products that our bodies normally keep in check are allowed to build up and cause havoc. It's a vicious cycle since oxidative stress can lead to even more inflammation.

If left uncontrolled, the damage induced by inflammation and oxidative stress can result in major health problems such as:

- High blood pressure
- Diabetes
- Cardiovascular disease
- Cancer
- Liver disease
- Kidney failure

This explains why nutritionists and doctors recommend consuming foods high in antioxidants, which fight oxidative stress and are an essential component of an anti-inflammatory diet.

How to Make Diet Changes to Reduce Inflammation

The most important thing is to restrict inflammation-causing meals, such as drinks, refined carbs, processed and packaged foods. "

Instead, we should consume a diet rich in healthier, natural sources of carbohydrates and fats, as well as the protein and fiber we require, such as fruits, vegetables, whole grains, legumes, and nuts, as well as enough of fatty fish and olive oil.

These are foods that contribute to insulin stabilization and a well-balanced omega-3 to omega-6 fat ratio, lowering the risk of inflammation. They are also unlikely to contribute to weight gain when ingested in suitable portions.

PART 4

The Potassium, Phosphorus, and Sodium Counter

L iving with kidney illness necessitates a thorough awareness of how food choices influence overall health. Maintaining kidney function requires a careful balance of potassium, phosphorus, and salt. This portion of our book attempts to empower kidney disease patients by providing a thorough meal list counter.

Controlling potassium levels is critical for those with renal disease who want to avoid problems like hyperkalemia. High-potassium foods like bananas and oranges should be consumed in moderation, whereas low-potassium foods like apples and berries give essential nutrients without raising potassium levels.

Controlling phosphorus consumption is critical to avoiding bone and cardiovascular problems caused by high amounts. This book encourages lean meats like chicken and turkey, as well as carbohydrates like white rice and quinoa, to provide low-phosphorus options for a balanced diet.

Controlling sodium levels is critical for controlling blood pressure and fluid retention. Low-sodium choices such as fresh veggies, unsalted nuts, and herbs allow people to enjoy savory meals without jeopardizing their kidney health. Reading labels and choosing low-sodium, homemade options is critical in sustaining heart health.

I hope you're having a good time with this book. If you require any clarification, please contact me at medlifeconsults@gmail.com *. As a token of* *appreciation, I humbly request that you leave a review on the website; this unique act of yours means the world to me as an independent publisher, and will assist me in tailoring my upcoming book to match your specific health needs.*

Below are specially crafted food list for optimizing your kidneys. Keep reading!

Low-Potassium Food List

Baked Foods:

1. White Bread (in moderation)
2. Plain Bagels
3. Unsalted Pretzels
4. White Cake
5. Vanilla Wafers
6. Angel Food Cake
7. Lemon Bars
8. Shortbread Cookies
9. Rice Cakes

10. Biscotti (without nuts)

11. Pound Cake

12. Ginger Snaps

13. Animal Crackers

14. Pita Bread (white)

15. Croissants (in moderation)

16. English Muffins

17. Rye Bread (in moderation)

18. Sponge Cake

19. Tortillas (corn)

20. Oatmeal Cookies (without nuts)

21. Donuts (in moderation)

22. Breadsticks

23. French Bread (in moderation)

24. Coffee Cake (in moderation)

25. Waffles (in moderation)

Beans and Lentils:

1. Lentils

2. Chickpeas (canned, rinsed)

3. Black Beans (canned, rinsed)

4. Navy Beans (dried, soaked, and boiled)

5. Great Northern Beans (canned, rinsed)

6. Pinto Beans (canned, rinsed)

7. Split Peas (dried, soaked, and boiled)

8. Black-eyed Peas (canned, rinsed)

9. Cannellini Beans (canned, rinsed)

10. Adzuki Beans (canned, rinsed)

11. Lima Beans (frozen, boiled)

12. Red Kidney Beans (canned, rinsed)

13. Butter Beans (canned, rinsed)

14. Cranberry Beans (dried, soaked, and boiled)

15. Garbanzo Beans (canned, rinsed)

16. Mung Beans (dried, soaked, and boiled)

17. Soybeans (edamame, boiled)

18. Black-eyed Peas (dried, soaked, and boiled)

19. Fava Beans (canned, rinsed)

20. Lentil Soup (homemade, low potassium ingredients)

21. Bean Burritos (homemade with low-potassium ingredients)

22. Refried Beans (low-potassium recipe)

23. Baked Beans (homemade with low-potassium ingredients)

24. Lentil Salad (low-potassium ingredients)

25. Bean Dip (low-potassium recipe)

Beverages:

1. Water

2. Herbal Tea (unsweetened)

3. Cranberry Juice (in moderation)

4. Apple Juice (in moderation)

5. Grape Juice (in moderation)

6. Lemonade (homemade with limited sugar)

7. Pineapple Juice (in moderation)

8. Pear Juice (in moderation)

9. Peach Nectar (in moderation)

10. Apricot Nectar (in moderation)

11. Mango Juice (in moderation)

12. Carrot Juice (in moderation)

13. Beet Juice (in moderation)

14. Cucumber Juice (in moderation)

15. Cherry Juice (in moderation)

16. Orange Juice (in moderation)

17. Tomato Juice (low-sodium)

18. Vegetable Juice (low-sodium)

19. Coconut Water (in moderation)

20. Sports Drinks (low potassium, low sodium)

21. Rice Milk (low potassium)

22. Almond Milk (low potassium)

23. Soy Milk (low potassium)

24. Hemp Milk (low potassium)

25. Cashew Milk (low potassium)

Breakfast Cereals:

1. Rice Cereal (low potassium)

2. Corn Flakes

3. Cream of Wheat

4. Rice Krispies

5. Puffed Rice

6. Bran Flakes

7. Cheerios

8. Wheat Chex

9. Corn Pops

10. Special K

11. Rice Chex

12. Kix

13. Shredded Wheat (original)

14. Rice Bran Cereal

15. Quaker Oats (original)

16. Oat Bran Cereal

17. Corn Bran Cereal

18. Farina

19. Wheat Germ Cereal

20. Grape-Nuts

21. All-Bran

22. Muesli (low potassium ingredients)

23. Granola (low potassium ingredients)

24. Oatmeal (in moderation)

25. Buckwheat Cereal (low potassium)

Dairy and Alternatives:

1. Almond Milk (low potassium)

2. Rice Milk

3. Unsalted Butter

4. Non-Dairy Creamer (low potassium)

5. Cream Cheese

6. Sour Cream (low-fat)

7. Cottage Cheese

8. Non-Dairy Yogurt (low potassium)

9. Ricotta Cheese

10. Goat Cheese

11. Gouda Cheese (low-fat)

12. Havarti Cheese (low-fat)

13. Mascarpone Cheese

14. Neufchâtel Cheese

15. Quark Cheese

16. String Cheese (low-fat)

17. Tofu (low potassium)

18. Vegan Cheese (low potassium)

19. Soy Yogurt (low potassium)

20. Hemp Milk (low potassium)

21. Cashew Cheese (low potassium)

22. Oat Milk (low potassium)

23. Flax Milk (low potassium)

24. Hazelnut Milk (low potassium)

25. Macadamia Milk (low potassium)

Dressing:

1. Olive Oil-based Dressing

2. Lemon Juice (for flavor)

3. Balsamic Vinegar

4. Italian Dressing (low-sodium)

5. Greek Yogurt Dressing (homemade)

6. Honey Mustard (homemade with limited salt)

7. Sesame Oil (in moderation)

8. Avocado Oil-based Dressing

9. Raspberry Vinaigrette

10. Tahini Dressing (low potassium)

11. Dijon Mustard Vinaigrette

12. Miso Dressing (low sodium)

13. Cilantro Lime Dressing

14. Apple Cider Vinegar (low potassium)

15. Pesto Sauce (low sodium)

16. Garlic Aioli (low sodium)

17. Mango Salsa (low sodium)

18. Pineapple Salsa (low sodium)

19. Tzatziki Sauce (low sodium)

20. Ranch Dressing (low potassium)

21. Thousand Island Dressing (low sodium)

22. Caesar Dressing (low potassium)

23. Blue Cheese Dressing (low sodium)

24. Poppyseed Dressing (low potassium)

25. Maple Dijon Dressing (low sodium)

Fats and Oils:

1. Olive Oil

2. Canola Oil

3. Avocado (in moderation)

4. Coconut Oil (in moderation)

5. Peanut Butter (low-sodium)

6. Sunflower Oil

7. Walnut Oil

8. Sesame Oil (in moderation)

9. Grapeseed Oil

10. Flaxseed Oil (in moderation)

11. Macadamia Nut Oil (in moderation)

12. Corn Oil (in moderation)

13. Safflower Oil (in moderation)

14. Hazelnut Oil (in moderation)

15. Hempseed Oil (in moderation)

16. Pistachio Oil (in moderation)

17. Almond Oil (in moderation)

18. Pecan Oil (in moderation)

19. Rice Bran Oil (in moderation)

20. MCT Oil (in moderation)

21. Pumpkin Seed Oil (in moderation)

22. Black Seed Oil (in moderation)

23. Soybean Oil (in moderation)

24. Duck Fat (in moderation)

25. Bacon Fat (in moderation)

These food selections above provide a varied selection across many cuisine categories while emphasizing kidney-friendly options.

Now that you have a dietary list, we have considered that certain patients would undoubtedly struggle to combine these food items in the proper proportion to make nutritious meals for their kidney function. With these considerations in mind, we have dedicated the next part of this book to making quick and easy renal-friendly dishes that will maximize your kidney function and keep you off surgeon's door!

Part 4

Renal-Friendly Recipes to Keep You off Your Surgeon's Door

Soups and stews

Recipe 1: **Vegetable Quinoa Soup**

Description: A comforting and nutritious soup loaded with vegetables and quinoa, perfect for a wholesome meal.

PREP TIME: 15 minutes
COOK TIME: 30 minutes
TOTAL TIME: 45 minutes

SERVINGS: 6

Ingredients:

- 1 cup quinoa, rinsed
- 1 tablespoon olive oil
- 1 onion, diced
- 2 cloves garlic, minced
- 3 carrots, peeled and diced
- 2 celery stalks, diced
- 1 bell pepper, diced
- 1 can (14 oz) diced tomatoes
- 6 cups low-sodium vegetable broth
- 2 teaspoons dried thyme
- Salt and pepper to taste
- Fresh parsley for garnish (optional)

Preparation:

1. **Prepare Quinoa**: In a saucepan, cook quinoa according to package instructions. Set aside.

2. **Sauté Vegetables**: In a medium sized pot, heat olive oil over medium heat. Add diced onion and garlic. Sauté until fragrant, about 2 minutes. Add carrots, celery, and bell pepper. Cook for an additional 5 minutes until vegetables begin to soften.

3. **Add Ingredients**: Pour in diced tomatoes (with their juices) and low-sodium vegetable broth. Stir in cooked quinoa and dried thyme. Season with salt and pepper to taste. Bring the soup to a boil.

4. **Simmer Soup**: Reduce heat to low, cover, and simmer for 20-25 minutes until the vegetables are tender and flavors are well combined.

5. **Serve**: Ladle the soup into bowls. Garnish with fresh parsley if desired. Serve hot and enjoy this hearty Vegetable Quinoa Soup!

Nutritional Information: (per serving - estimated)

- Calories: 220
- Protein: 7g
- Carbohydrates: 35g
- Fiber: 6g
- Fat: 6g

Recipe 2: **Lentil Stew**

Description: A comforting and protein-packed stew made with lentils and flavorful spices.

PREP TIME: 10 minutes
COOK TIME: 40 minutes
TOTAL TIME: 50 minutes
SERVINGS: 4

Ingredients:

- 1 cup properly dried green or brown lentils, rinsed
- 2 tablespoons olive oil
- 1 onion, chopped
- 3 cloves garlic, minced
- 2 carrots, diced
- 2 celery stalks, diced
- 1 can (14 oz) diced tomatoes
- 4 cups low-sodium vegetable broth
- 1 teaspoon ground cumin
- 1 teaspoon paprika
- Salt and pepper to taste
- Fresh parsley for garnish (optional)

Instructions:

1. **Cook Lentils:** In a pot, bring 2 cups of water to a boil. Add rinsed lentils and cook for 15-20 minutes until tender. Sieve out any excess water and set aside.

2. **Sauté Aromatics:** In a large pot, heat olive oil over medium heat. Add chopped onion and minced garlic. Sauté until translucent, about 3 minutes. Add diced carrots and celery. Cook for an additional 5 minutes.

3. **Combine Ingredients:** Pour in diced tomatoes (with their juices), low-sodium vegetable broth, cooked lentils, ground cumin, paprika, salt, and pepper. Bring the mixture to a simmer.

4. **Simmer Stew:** Reduce heat to low, cover, and simmer for 20-25 minutes, allowing the flavors to meld and the stew to thicken.

5. **Serve:** Ladle the lentil stew into bowls. Garnish with fresh parsley if desired. Serve hot and relish this delightful Lentil Stew!

Nutritional Information: (per serving - estimated)

- Calories: 280
- Protein: 15g
- Carbohydrates: 45g
- Fiber: 12g
- Fat: 6g

Recipe 3: **Chicken and Vegetable Broth**

Description: A comforting and flavorful broth combining chicken and assorted vegetables.

PREP TIME: 10 minutes
COOK TIME: 1 hour
TOTAL TIME: 1 hour 10 minutes
SERVINGS: 6

Ingredients:

- 1 whole chicken (about 3-4 lbs), cut into pieces
- 8 cups water

- 2 carrots, chopped
- 2 celery stalks, chopped
- 1 onion, quartered
- 2 cloves garlic, smashed
- 1 bay leaf
- 1 teaspoon whole peppercorns
- Salt to taste
- Fresh parsley for garnish (optional)

Instructions:

1. **Prepare Chicken Broth:** In a large pot, combine chicken pieces, water, chopped carrots, celery, onion, smashed garlic, bay leaf, whole peppercorns, and a pinch of salt. Bring to a boil.

2. **Simmer Broth:** Reduce heat to low, cover, and simmer for about 1 hour. Skim off any foam that rises to the surface occasionally.

3. **Strain Broth:** Once the broth is flavorful and the chicken is cooked through, remove the chicken pieces and strain the broth through a fine-mesh sieve. Discard the solids.

4. **Serve:** Use the chicken and vegetable broth as a base for soups or enjoy it as a comforting and nourishing broth on its own. Garnish with fresh parsley if desired.

Nutritional Information: (per serving - estimated)

- Calories: 120
- Protein: 18g
- Carbohydrates: 2g
- Fiber: 0.5g
- Fat: 5g

Recipe 4: **Minestrone Soup**

Description: A hearty Italian soup loaded with vegetables, beans, and pasta.

PREP TIME: 15 minutes
COOK TIME: 30 minutes
TOTAL TIME: 45 minutes
SERVINGS: 6

Ingredients:
- 2 tablespoons olive oil
- 1 onion, diced
- 2 cloves garlic, minced
- 2 carrots, diced
- 2 celery stalks, diced
- 1 can (14 oz) diced tomatoes
- 6 cups low-sodium vegetable broth
- 1 can (14 oz) kidney beans, drained and rinsed
- 1 cup small pasta (ditalini or elbow)

- 2 cups chopped spinach or kale
- 1 teaspoon dried basil
- Salt and pepper to taste
- Grated Parmesan cheese for serving (optional)

Preparation:

1. **Sauté Vegetables:** In a large pot, heat olive oil over medium heat. Add diced onion and minced garlic. Sauté until fragrant, about 2 minutes. Add diced carrots and celery. Cook for an additional 5 minutes until vegetables begin to soften.

2. **Add Ingredients:** Pour in diced tomatoes (with their juices), low-sodium vegetable broth, drained kidney beans, and dried basil. Bring the soup to a boil.

3. **Simmer Soup:** Reduce heat to low, cover, and simmer for 15 minutes. Add small pasta and chopped

spinach or kale. Continue to simmer for an additional 10 minutes until the pasta is al dente.

4. **Season and Serve:** Finally, season your soup with salt and pepper to taste. Ladle into bowls and serve hot. Optionally, top with grated Parmesan cheese before serving.

Nutritional Information: (per serving - estimated)

- Calories: 250
- Protein: 10g
- Carbohydrates: 40g
- Fiber: 8g
- Fat: 6g

Snacks and Appetizers

Recipe 5: **Rice Cake with Cottage Cheese**

Description: A simple and light snack featuring rice cakes topped with creamy cottage cheese.

PREP TIME: 5 minutes
COOK TIME: 0 minutes
TOTAL TIME: 5 minutes
SERVINGS: 2

Ingredients:
- 2 rice cakes (low-sodium, if available)
- 1/2 cup low-sodium cottage cheese
- 1 tablespoon chopped chives or scallions (optional)
- Black pepper to taste

Preparation:

1. **Assemble:** Place rice cakes on a serving plate. Spread a generous dollop of low-sodium cottage cheese on each rice cake.

2. **Garnish:** Sprinkle chopped chives or scallions on top of the cottage cheese. Add a dash of black pepper for flavor.

Nutritional Information: (per serving - estimated)

- Calories: 110
- Protein: 7g
- Carbohydrates: 14g
- Fiber: 1g
- Fat: 3g
- Potassium: 90mg
- Phosphorus: 80mg
- Sodium: 120mg

Recipe 6: **Mixed Nuts and Seeds**

Description: A nutrient-dense mix of assorted nuts and seeds for a satisfying and healthy snack.

PREP TIME: 5 minutes
COOK TIME: 0 minutes
TOTAL TIME: 5 minutes
SERVINGS: 4

Ingredients:

- 1/2 cup almonds (unsalted)
- 1/2 cup walnuts (unsalted)
- 1/4 cup pumpkin seeds
- 1/4 cup sunflower seeds
- 1/4 teaspoon salt (optional, low-sodium if preferred)
- 1/2 teaspoon ground cinnamon (optional)

Preparation:

1. **Combine Nuts and Seeds**: In a bowl, mix together almonds, walnuts, pumpkin seeds, and sunflower seeds. Add a sprinkle of salt if desired (choose low-sodium) and a touch of ground cinnamon for added flavor.

2. **Portion and Serve:** Divide the mixed nuts and seeds into individual servings or store in an airtight container for a ready-to-go healthy snack.

Nutritional Information: (per serving – estimated)

- Calories: 180
- Protein: 6g
- Carbohydrates: 5g
- Fiber: 3g
- Fat: 15g
- Potassium: 160mg
- Phosphorus: 110mg
- Sodium: 75mg

Recipe 7: **Hummus with Veggies**

Description: Creamy hummus paired with assorted fresh vegetables makes for a delightful and nutritious snack.

PREP TIME: 10 minutes
COOK TIME: 0 minutes
TOTAL TIME: 10 minutes
SERVINGS: 4

Ingredients:

- 1 can (15 oz) chickpeas, drained and rinsed
- 3 tablespoons tahini
- 2 tablespoons lemon juice
- 2 cloves garlic, minced
- 2 tablespoons olive oil
- Salt and pepper to taste

- Assorted fresh vegetables (carrots, cucumbers, bell peppers) for dipping

Preparation:

1. **Prepare Hummus:** In a food processor, blend chickpeas, tahini, lemon juice, minced garlic, olive oil, salt, and pepper until smooth and creamy. If needed, adjust consistency by adding a little water.

2. **Serve:** Transfer the hummus to a serving bowl. Arrange assorted fresh vegetables around the hummus for dipping.

Nutritional Information: (per serving - estimated)

- Calories: 180
- Protein: 6g
- Carbohydrates: 20g
- Fiber: 6g
- Fat: 9g

Recipe 8: **Guacamole with Baked Tortilla Chips**

Description: A classic guacamole paired with homemade baked tortilla chips for a satisfying snack.

PREP TIME: 15 minutes
COOK TIME: 10 minutes
TOTAL TIME: 25 minutes
SERVINGS: 4

Ingredients:

- 2 ripe avocados
- 1 tomato, diced
- 1/4 cup red onion, finely chopped
- 2 tablespoons fresh cilantro, chopped
- 1 lime, juiced
- Salt and pepper to taste
- 4 corn tortillas

Instructions:

1. **Prepare Guacamole:** In a bowl, mash the ripe avocados. Add diced tomato, chopped red onion, chopped cilantro, lime juice, salt, and pepper. Mix until well combined.

2. **Bake Tortilla Chips:** Preheat oven to 350°F (175°C). Cut each corn tortilla into wedges. Arrange the wedges on a baking sheet. Bake for 8-10 minutes until crispy.

3. **Serve:** Place the guacamole in a serving bowl and serve alongside the baked tortilla chips.

Nutritional Information: (per serving - estimated)
- Calories: 180
- Protein: 3g
- Carbohydrates: 20g
- Fiber: 6g

- Fat: 11g

Mains

Recipe 9: **Baked Lemon Herb Chicken**

Description: Tender chicken breasts baked with zesty lemon and aromatic herbs for a flavorful and healthy main course.

PREP TIME: 10 minutes
COOK TIME: 25 minutes
TOTAL TIME: 35 minutes
SERVINGS: 4

Ingredients:

- 4 boneless, skinless chicken breasts
- 2 tablespoons olive oil
- 2 cloves garlic, minced
- 1 teaspoon dried thyme

- 1 teaspoon dried rosemary
- Zest of 1 lemon
- Juice of 1 lemon
- Salt and pepper to taste
- Fresh parsley for garnish (optional)

Preparation:

1. **Preheat Oven:** Preheat oven to 400°F (200°C).

2. **Prepare Chicken:** Place chicken breasts in a baking dish. Drizzle olive oil over the chicken. Add minced garlic, dried thyme, dried rosemary, lemon zest, and lemon juice. Rub the mixture evenly over the chicken. Season with salt and pepper.

3. **Bake Chicken:** Bake in the preheated oven for 20-25 minutes or until the chicken is cooked through and juices run clear.

4. **Serve:** Remove from the oven and let it rest for a few minutes. Garnish with fresh parsley if desired. Serve this delightful Baked Lemon Herb Chicken hot.

Nutritional Information: (per serving - estimated)

- Calories: 240
- Protein: 28g
- Carbohydrates: 2g
- Fiber: 0.5g
- Fat: 13g
- Potassium: 280mg
- Phosphorus: 200mg
- Sodium: 110mg

Recipe 10: **Grilled Salmon with Herbs**

Description: Succulent salmon fillets grilled with a blend of herbs for a tasty and nutritious main dish.

PREP TIME: 10 minutes

COOK TIME: 10 minutes

TOTAL TIME: 20 minutes

SERVINGS: 4

Ingredients:

- 4 skin -on, salmon fillets (6 oz each)

- 2 tablespoons olive oil

- 1 tablespoon fresh dill, chopped

- 1 tablespoon fresh parsley, chopped

- 1 tablespoon fresh thyme leaves

- 1 lemon, sliced

- Salt and pepper to taste

Preparation:

1. **Preheat Grill:** Preheat the grill to medium-high heat.

2. **Prepare Salmon**: Brush salmon fillets with olive oil. Sprinkle chopped fresh dill, parsley, and thyme over the fillets. Season with salt and pepper. Place lemon slices on top of the fillets.

3. **Grill Salmon**: Place the seasoned salmon fillets skin-side down on the grill. Grill each side for about 4-5 minutes, or until the salmon easily flakes with a fork.

4. **Serve**: Remove from the grill and transfer to a serving platter. Serve this delectable Grilled Salmon with Herbs alongside your favorite side dishes.

Nutritional Information: (per serving - estimated)

- Calories: 300
- Protein: 34g
- Carbohydrates: 1g
- Fiber: 0.5g
- Fat: 18g
- Potassium: 450mg
- Phosphorus: 350mg
- Sodium: 75mg

Recipe 11: **Turkey Stir-Fry**

Description: A flavorful and protein-packed stir-fry featuring lean turkey and assorted vegetables.

PREP TIME: 15 minutes
COOK TIME: 15 minutes
TOTAL TIME: 30 minutes
SERVINGS: 4

Ingredients:
- 1 lb turkey breast, thinly sliced
- 2 tablespoons low-sodium soy sauce
- 2 tablespoons olive oil
- 1 onion, sliced
- 2 bell peppers (assorted colors), sliced
- 1 cup snow peas, trimmed
- 2 cloves garlic, minced
- 1 teaspoon ginger, minced
- Salt and pepper to taste

- Sesame seeds for garnish (optional)
- Cooked brown rice for serving (optional)

Preparation:

1. **Marinate Turkey**: In a bowl, marinate thinly sliced turkey breast in low-sodium soy sauce for 10 minutes.

2. **Stir-Fry Turkey**: Heat olive oil in a large skillet or wok over medium-high heat. Add marinated turkey and cook until browned, about 5-6 minutes. Take off turkey from the skillet and set aside.

3. **Cook Vegetables**: In the same skillet, add sliced onion, bell peppers, snow peas, minced garlic, and minced ginger. Stir-fry for about 5 minutes until vegetables are tender yet crisp.

4. **Combine Ingredients**: Return the cooked turkey to the skillet. Toss everything together and cook for an

additional 2-3 minutes until heated through. To taste, season with salt and pepper.

5. **Serve:** Serve this delicious Turkey Stir-Fry garnished with sesame seeds, if desired. Pair with cooked brown rice if desired for a complete meal.

Nutritional Information: (per serving - estimated)

- Calories: 250
- Protein: 28g
- Carbohydrates: 10g
- Fiber: 3g
- Fat: 12g
- Potassium: 350mg
- Phosphorus: 250mg
- Sodium: 350mg

Recipe 12: Eggplant Parmesan (Baked)

Description: A healthier version of the classic Eggplant Parmesan, baked to golden perfection without sacrificing flavor.

PREP TIME: 25 minutes
COOK TIME: 40 minutes
TOTAL TIME: 1 hour 5 minutes
SERVINGS: 6

Ingredients:
- 2 large eggplants, sliced into 1/4-inch rounds
- 2 eggs, beaten
- 1 cup breadcrumbs (whole-grain or gluten-free)
- 1/2 cup grated Parmesan cheese (low-sodium if available)
- 2 cups marinara sauce (low-sodium)
- 1 cup shredded mozzarella cheese (low-fat if preferred)

- Fresh basil leaves for garnish (optional)

Preparation:

1. **Prepare Eggplant Slices:** Preheat oven to 375°F (190°C). Line a baking sheet with parchment paper. Dip eggplant slices into beaten eggs, then coat both sides with breadcrumbs mixed with grated Parmesan cheese. Place coated slices on the baking sheet. Bake for 25-30 minutes until golden brown.

2. **Assemble Eggplant Parmesan:** In a baking dish, spread a thin layer of marinara sauce. Place half of the baked eggplant slices over the sauce. Add another layer of marinara sauce and sprinkle shredded mozzarella cheese on top. Redo the layers with the remaining eggplant, marinara sauce, and mozzarella cheese.

3. **Bake:** Cover the baking dish with foil and bake for an additional 15-20 minutes or until the cheese is melted and bubbly.

4. **Serve:** Garnish with fresh basil leaves if desired. Serve this delightful Baked Eggplant Parmesan as a comforting main dish.

Nutritional Information: (per serving - estimated)

- Calories: 220
- Protein: 12g
- Carbohydrates: 25g
- Fiber: 7g
- Fat: 8g
- Potassium: 320mg
- Phosphorus: 170mg
- Sodium: 320mg

Side Dishes

Recipe 13: **Steamed Asparagus with Lemon**

Description: A simple yet flavorful side dish featuring tender asparagus spears enhanced with zesty lemon.

PREP TIME: 5 minutes
COOK TIME: 5 minutes
TOTAL TIME: 10 minutes
SERVINGS: 4

Ingredients:

- 1 bunch asparagus, ends trimmed
- Zest of 1 lemon
- 1 tablespoon olive oil
- Salt and pepper to taste
- Lemon wedges for garnish (optional)

Preparation:

1. **Prepare Asparagus:** Fill a large skillet or pot with an inch of water. Bring the water to a boil. Add trimmed asparagus spears to a steamer basket or directly into the pot. Cover and steam for 3-5 minutes until the asparagus is tender yet crisp.

2. **Enhance Flavors:** In a bowl, mix together lemon zest, olive oil, salt, and pepper.

3. **Season Asparagus:** Remove the steamed asparagus from the heat and drizzle the lemon-infused olive oil mixture over the spears. Toss gently to coat evenly.

4. **Serve:** Transfer the steamed asparagus to a serving dish. Garnish with lemon wedges if desired. Serve this delightful Steamed Asparagus with Lemon as a refreshing side.

Nutritional Information: (per serving - estimated)

- Calories: 40
- Protein: 2g
- Carbohydrates: 4g
- Fiber: 2g
- Fat: 3g
- Potassium: 200mg
- Phosphorus: 40mg
- Sodium: 5mg

Recipe 14: **Garlic Mashed Cauliflower**

Description: A creamy and flavorful alternative to mashed potatoes using cauliflower with a hint of garlic.

PREP TIME: 10 minutes
COOK TIME: 15 minutes
TOTAL TIME: 25 minutes
SERVINGS: 4

Ingredients:

- 1 head cauliflower, chopped into florets
- 2 cloves garlic, minced
- 2 tablespoons unsalted butter (or olive oil for a healthier option)
- Salt and pepper to taste
- Chopped fresh parsley for garnish (optional)

Preparation:

1. **Cook Cauliflower:** In a pot of boiling water, cook cauliflower florets and minced garlic for 10-12 minutes until tender.

2. **Mash Cauliflower:** Drain the cooked cauliflower and transfer to a large bowl. Using a potato masher or immersion blender mash the cauliflower until smooth.

Add butter (or olive oil), salt, and pepper. Continue mashing process until desired consistency is achieved.

3. **Season and Serve:** Adjust seasoning as needed. Garnish with chopped fresh parsley if desired. Serve this delicious Garlic Mashed Cauliflower as a delightful side dish.

Nutritional Information: (per serving - estimated)

- Calories: 70
- Protein: 3g
- Carbohydrates: 7g
- Fiber: 3g
- Fat: 4g
- Potassium: 320mg
- Phosphorus: 80mg
- Sodium: 30mg

Recipe 15: **Quinoa Pilaf**

Description: A nutritious and flavorful pilaf made with quinoa, mixed vegetables, and aromatic spices.

PREP TIME: 10 minutes
COOK TIME: 20 minutes
TOTAL TIME: 30 minutes
SERVINGS: 4

Ingredients:

- 1 cup quinoa, rinsed
- 2 cups low-sodium vegetable broth
- 1 tablespoon olive oil
- 1 small onion, finely chopped
- 2 cloves garlic, minced
- 1 carrot, diced
- 1 bell pepper (any color), diced
- 1 teaspoon ground cumin
- 1 teaspoon paprika

- Salt and pepper to taste

- Chopped fresh parsley for garnish (optional)

Preparation:

1. **Prepare Quinoa:** In a pot, bring vegetable broth to a boil. Add rinsed quinoa, cover, and simmer for 15-20 minutes until quinoa is cooked and liquid is absorbed.

2. **Sauté Vegetables:** In a skillet, heat olive oil over medium heat. Add finely chopped onion, minced garlic, diced carrot, and diced bell pepper. Sauté vegetables for 5-7 minutes until tender.

3. **Combine Ingredients:** Add cooked quinoa to the skillet with sautéed vegetables. Sprinkle ground cumin, paprika, salt, and pepper. Stir well to combine all ingredients.

4. **Serve:** Transfer the Quinoa Pilaf to a serving dish. Garnish with chopped fresh parsley if desired. Serve this flavorful pilaf as a wholesome side dish.

Nutritional Information: (per serving - estimated)

- Calories: 220
- Protein: 6g
- Carbohydrates: 35g
- Fiber: 5g
- Fat: 6g
- Potassium: 300mg
- Phosphorus: 150mg
- Sodium: 50mg

Recipe 16: **Roasted Brussels Sprouts**

Description: Simple yet delicious roasted Brussels sprouts seasoned with olive oil and spices for a delightful side dish.

PREP TIME: 10 minutes

COOK TIME: 25 minutes

TOTAL TIME: 35 minutes

SERVINGS: 4

Ingredients:

- 1 lb Brussels sprouts, halved and trimmed
- 2 tablespoons olive oil
- 2 cloves garlic, minced
- Salt and pepper to taste
- 1 tablespoon balsamic vinegar (optional)
- Grated Parmesan cheese for garnish (optional)

Preparation:

1. **Preheat Oven**: Preheat oven to 400°F (200°C).

2. **Prepare Brussels Sprouts**: Place trimmed and halved Brussels sprouts on a baking sheet. Drizzle with

olive oil and minced garlic. Season with salt and pepper. Toss to coat evenly.

3. **Roast Brussels Sprouts:** Roast in the preheated oven for 20-25 minutes until Brussels sprouts are golden brown and tender, stirring halfway through.

4. **Enhance Flavors:** Drizzle with balsamic vinegar for added flavor (optional) and sprinkle with grated Parmesan cheese if desired.

5. **Serve:** Transfer the Roasted Brussels Sprouts to a serving dish. Serve this delightful side dish hot.

Nutritional Information: (per serving - estimated)
- Calories: 90
- Protein: 4g
- Carbohydrates: 10g
- Fiber: 4g
- Fat: 5g

- Potassium: 320mg
- Phosphorus: 100mg
- Sodium: 30mg

Salads

Recipe 17: **Greek Salad**

Description: A refreshing and classic Greek salad featuring fresh vegetables, feta cheese, olives, and a tangy vinaigrette.

PREP TIME: 15 minutes
COOK TIME: 0 minutes
TOTAL TIME: 15 minutes
SERVINGS: 4

Ingredients:
- 2 cups cherry tomatoes, halved

- 1 cucumber, diced
- 1 red onion, thinly sliced
- 1 green bell pepper, diced
- 1/2 cup Kalamata olives, pitted
- 1/2 cup crumbled feta cheese (low-fat if preferred)
- 2 tablespoons olive oil
- 1 tablespoon red wine vinegar
- 1 teaspoon dried oregano
- Salt and pepper to taste
- Fresh parsley for garnish (optional)

Instructions:

1. **Prepare Vegetables:** In a large bowl, combine halved cherry tomatoes, diced cucumber, thinly sliced red onion, diced green bell pepper, and Kalamata olives.

2. **Add Feta Cheese:** Sprinkle crumbled feta cheese over the vegetables.

3. **Make Vinaigrette:** In a small bowl, whisk together olive oil, red wine vinegar, dried oregano, salt, and pepper.

4. **Dress Salad:** Drizzle the vinaigrette over the salad and toss gently to combine all ingredients.

5. **Garnish and Serve:** Garnish with fresh parsley if desired. Serve this delightful Greek Salad as a refreshing side or main dish.

Nutritional Information: (per serving - estimated)

- Calories: 150
- Protein: 4g
- Carbohydrates: 10g
- Fiber: 3g
- Fat: 11g
- Potassium: 320mg
- Phosphorus: 90mg

- Sodium: 350mg

Recipe 18: **Spinach and Strawberry Salad**

Description: A vibrant salad combining fresh spinach, sweet strawberries, and a light vinaigrette for a burst of flavors.

PREP TIME: 10 minutes
COOK TIME: 0 minutes
TOTAL TIME: 10 minutes
SERVINGS: 4

Ingredients:

- 6 cups fresh spinach leaves, washed and dried
- 2 cups fresh strawberries, sliced
- 1/4 cup sliced almonds
- 2 tablespoons balsamic vinegar
- 1 tablespoon olive oil

- 1 teaspoon honey or maple syrup
- Salt and pepper to taste

Instructions:

1. **Prepare Salad Base:** In a large bowl, combine fresh spinach leaves and sliced strawberries.

2. **Toast Almonds:** In a dry skillet over medium heat, toast sliced almonds until lightly golden and fragrant, about 2-3 minutes. Remove from heat.

3. **Make Vinaigrette:** In a small bowl, whisk together balsamic vinegar, olive oil, honey (or maple syrup), salt, and pepper to create the dressing.

4. **Assemble Salad:** Sprinkle toasted almonds over the spinach and strawberry mixture. Drizzle the vinaigrette over the salad and toss gently to coat.

5. **Serve:** Serve this vibrant Spinach and Strawberry Salad as a refreshing side or add grilled chicken for a complete meal.

Nutritional Information: (per serving - estimated)
- Calories: 110
- Protein: 3g
- Carbohydrates: 11g
- Fiber: 4g
- Fat: 7g
- Potassium: 350mg
- Phosphorus: 80mg
- -Sodium: 50mg

Recipe 19: **Cucumber and Tomato Salad**

Description: A light and refreshing salad combining crisp cucumbers, juicy tomatoes, and a simple vinaigrette.

PREP TIME: 10 minutes

COOK TIME: 0 minutes

TOTAL TIME: 10 minutes

SERVINGS: 4

Ingredients:

- 2 cucumbers, thinly sliced
- 2 tomatoes, diced
- 1/4 red onion, thinly sliced
- 2 tbs chopped fresh basil or parsley
- 2 tablespoons olive oil
- 1 tablespoon white wine vinegar or lemon juice
- 1 teaspoon honey or sugar (optional)
- Salt and pepper to taste

Instructions:

1. **Prepare Vegetables**: In a large bowl, combine thinly sliced cucumbers, diced tomatoes, thinly sliced

red onion, and chopped fresh parsley or basil.

2. **Make Vinaigrette:** In a small bowl, whisk together olive oil, white wine vinegar (or lemon juice), honey (or sugar, if using), salt, and pepper to create the dressing.

3. **Dress Salad:** Drizzle the vinaigrette over the cucumber and tomato mixture. Toss with ease to coat all ingredients evenly.

4. **Serve:** Serve this light and refreshing Cucumber and Tomato Salad as a delightful side or a quick snack.

Nutritional Information: (per serving - estimated)
- Calories: 80
- Protein: 2g
- Carbohydrates: 7g
- Fiber: 2g
- Fat: 6g

- Potassium: 260mg
- Phosphorus: 40mg
- Sodium: 10mg

Recipe 20: **Bean Salad**

Description: A flavorful and protein-packed salad made with assorted beans and a tangy dressing.

PREP TIME: 15 minutes
COOK TIME: 0 minutes
TOTAL TIME: 15 minutes
SERVINGS: 4

Ingredients:

- 1 can (15 oz) rinsed and sieved kidney beans
- 1 can (15 oz) rinsed and sieved chickpeas (garbanzo beans)

- 1 can (15 oz) rinsed and sieved black beans
- 1 diced red bell pepper - 1/2 finely chopped red onion - 1/4 cup chopped fresh cilantro or parsley - 2 tablespoons olive oil - 2 teaspoons red wine vinegar or apple cider vinegar
- 1 teaspoon honey or maple syrup
- 1 teaspoon ground cumin
- Salt and pepper to taste

Instructions:

1. **Prepare Beans:** In a large bowl, combine kidney beans, chickpeas, black beans, diced red bell pepper, finely chopped red onion, and chopped fresh cilantro or parsley.

2. **Make Dressing:** In a small bowl, whisk together olive oil, red wine vinegar (or apple cider vinegar),

honey (or maple syrup), ground cumin, salt, and pepper to create the dressing.

3. **Dress Salad:** Pour the dressing over the bean mixture. Toss gently to coat all ingredients with the dressing.

4. **Serve:** Serve this protein-rich and flavorful Bean Salad as a satisfying side dish or a standalone meal.

Nutritional Information: (per serving - estimated)

- Calories: 270
- Protein: 13g
- Carbohydrates: 38g
- Fiber: 11g
- Fat: 8g
- Potassium: 600mg
- Phosphorus: 200mg
- Sodium: 240mg

Dear readers, we hope you enjoyed the wide variety of kidney-friendly recipes in this book. We appreciate your culinary trip through these flavors, and we sincerely hope you find these recipes useful in managing your nutritional demands.

We gladly invite you to leave a review on our website to share your experience. Your input is extremely valuable since it drives us to respond to your specific needs through more customized books. Your feedback helps us create resources that are even more tailored to your needs.

Furthermore, we are pleased to inform that our book contains a supplementary section devoted to giving useful resources. This area tries to provide helpful materials to help you on your road to recovery and better health.

Thank you for joining us on this culinary adventure. Your feedback, ideas, and suggestions motivate us to keep providing content that is relevant to you.

I wish you good health and tasty meals.

Bonus 1

Effective Meal Planning Tips for Kidney Disease

Meal planning allows you to make better dietary choices and simplifies grocery shopping. It's also a great approach to boost your health if you have chronic kidney disease (CKD). By eating healthily every day, you may help yourself feel your best by choosing the right meals and monitoring your nutrition. When you learn how to design your balanced kidney disease meal plan, creating your kidney-friendly grocery list will be a piece of cake. Below are healthy steps to plan your Meals.

1. Understand your kidney health requirements.

When you have CKD, your kidneys do not balance the levels of nutrients and waste in your body as well as they should. You may help your kidneys by paying attention to which nutrients you consume and keeping track of your portions.

Every person has different dietary demands, and these needs may alter based on your stage of renal disease and how it is managed. For example, if you're on dialysis, you may need to watch your fluid consumption and increase your protein intake. If you have additional health issues, such as diabetes or heart disease, you'll need to incorporate those requirements into your diet as well. If you work with a nutritionist, they can assist you in developing a customized kidney disease meal plan that promotes your overall health. If you aren't visiting a dietician, talk to your doctor about meal planning.

2. Keep track of your minerals

If you have CKD, there are a few nutrients you should pay particular attention to. Here are some things to keep in mind while selecting meals for people with kidney disease:

Remove the salt by shaking it off. Healthy kidneys control your body's sodium and fluid levels, but if you have CKD, you'll need to aid support this process by limiting your sodium consumption.

Reduce your phosphorous consumption. Phosphorus buildup can be damaging to your bones and heart health if you have CKD. It occurs naturally in many foods and is sometimes added as a preservative, so read the nutrition label carefully and look for words beginning with "phos-."

Consume low-potassium foods. Potassium is essential for good health, but with CKD, your kidneys struggle to keep this vitamin in check. Excess potassium can create problems with your heart and nerves.

Proteins should be chosen with care. Protein, in moderation, maintains muscles strong and healthy.

Choose high-quality proteins like fish or poultry to reduce waste buildup, or try plant-based proteins to put less strain on your kidneys. It has been demonstrated that eating beans, tofu, almonds, and other plant-based proteins can help reduce the progression of renal disease and keep patients with CKD healthier for longer.

3. Understand how to read nutrition labels.

Eating fresh fruits, veggies, and meats is always a good idea, but you can also make kidney-friendly choices when purchasing packaged items. Packaged foods include nutrition labels that list the vitamins, minerals, fats, and calories in each serving. The percent daily value (% DV) indicates how much each serving adds to your daily diet (based on 2,000 calories). To keep your kidney disease meal planning on track, keep an eye on the% DV.

To keep your kidneys happy, strive for the following %DV with each serving:

- More than 10% DV for dietary fiber
- Saturated fat — less than 10% of the daily value
- There is no trans fat, and the sodium content is less than 10% of the DV.
- Sugars added — less than 10% DV

Also, patients with kidney illness should avoid items marked "phos-" on the label.

4. Divide your plate

The key to eating healthy, whether you're choosing meals for kidney illness or not, is to keep track of your servings. Take note of the serving size mentioned on the packaging. One serving may not be the same as how much you consume.

Remember that if you eat two serving sizes, all of the nutrients and %DV will double.

Here are some helpful hints for calculating portion sizes:

- 3-5 ounces of protein is around the size of your palm.
- 1/2 cup of fruits and vegetables is the quantity that might fit in the palm of your hand.
- 1 cup breads and grains is around the size of your fist.

5. Eat kidney-friendly meals all day.

Because your kidneys operate around the clock, it's critical to commit to eating healthy at every meal. Breakfast, lunch, snacks, and dinner all contribute to your overall health, especially on holidays and when dining out. Consider all of the varied foods you consume throughout the day and make a strategy to eat wisely at each meal.

Begin your day off right with a high-protein breakfast. This will help you control your hunger and reduce mindless snacking.

A well-balanced lunch will keep your renal disease diet on track. Replace salt with strong flavors such as citrus, spices, and fresh herbs.

You can still eat delectable foods if you have chronic renal disease. You may even prepare your favorite dishes in a kidney-friendly manner.

If you're ready for dessert, remember to watch your quantities and limit your intake of processed foods. For a nutritious boost, try adding fresh fruits, veggies, and grains.

Bonus 2

A 30-Day Kidney Disease Meal Plan

Below is a 30-day meal plan adapted for people with kidney illness, with a focus on protein-rich breakfasts, balanced lunches, kidney-friendly adaptations of favorite dinners, and mindful dessert options:

Day 1:

Breakfast: Scrambled eggs with spinach and mushrooms
Lunch: Grilled chicken salad with mixed greens
Dinner: Baked lemon herb salmon with steamed asparagus
Dessert: Fresh fruit salad

Day 2:

Breakfast: Greek yogurt parfait with berries and almonds
Lunch: Quinoa pilaf with roasted vegetables
Dinner: Turkey stir-fry with low-sodium soy sauce
Dessert: Baked apple slices with cinnamon

Day 3:

Breakfast: Cottage cheese with pineapple and walnuts
Lunch: Eggplant parmesan (baked) with a side salad
Dinner: Lentil stew with whole-grain bread
Dessert: Frozen grapes

Day 4:

Breakfast: Oatmeal with sliced banana and almond butter

Lunch: Spinach and strawberry salad with grilled chicken

Dinner: Baked lemon herb chicken with garlic mashed cauliflower

Dessert: Chia seed pudding with mixed berries

Day 5:

Breakfast: Smoked salmon and avocado on whole-grain toast

Lunch: Bean salad with bell peppers and herbs

Dinner: Grilled shrimp skewers with quinoa

Dessert: Greek yogurt with honey and sliced peaches

Day 6:

Breakfast: Spinach and feta omelet

Lunch: Cucumber and tomato salad with grilled tofu

Dinner: Roasted Brussels sprouts with baked cod

Dessert: Watermelon slices

Day 7:

Breakfast: Protein smoothie with kale, banana, and almond milk

Lunch: Hummus with veggie sticks and whole-grain crackers

Dinner: Chicken and vegetable broth with whole-grain bread

Dessert: Mango sorbet

Day 8:

Breakfast: Cottage cheese pancakes with fresh berries

Lunch: Tuna salad sandwich on whole-grain bread

Dinner: Baked herb-crusted tofu with quinoa and steamed broccoli

Dessert: Baked pear with a sprinkle of cinnamon

Day 9:

Breakfast: Breakfast burrito with scrambled eggs, black beans, and salsa

Lunch: Greek salad with grilled shrimp

Dinner: Turkey chili with kidney beans and a side of brown rice

Dessert: Sliced strawberries with a dollop of whipped cream (in moderation)

Day 10:

Breakfast: Whole-grain toast with almond butter and sliced apple

Lunch: Chicken Caesar salad with a light dressing

Dinner: Baked halibut with roasted vegetables

Dessert: Yogurt parfait with granola and mixed fruit

Day 11:

Breakfast: Spinach and mushroom frittata

Lunch: Lentil soup with whole-grain crackers

Dinner: Stir-fried tofu with mixed vegetables and brown rice

Dessert: Banana "nice cream" made with frozen bananas

Day 12:

Breakfast: Overnight oats with chia seeds and mixed berries

Lunch: Caprese salad with grilled chicken

Dinner: Baked turkey meatballs with zucchini noodles

Dessert: Melon skewers

Day 13:

Breakfast: Breakfast quinoa with cinnamon and raisins
Lunch: Mixed bean salad with bell peppers and vinaigrette
Dinner: Grilled swordfish with quinoa pilaf and roasted asparagus
Dessert: Apple slices dipped in Greek yogurt

Day 14:

Breakfast: Smoothie bowl with spinach, banana, and almond milk topped with nuts and seeds
Lunch: Vegetable stir-fry with tofu
Dinner: Chicken and vegetable broth with whole-grain bread
Dessert: Mixed fruit salad with a drizzle of honey

Day 15:

Breakfast: Greek yogurt with honey and mixed nuts
Lunch: Spinach and strawberry salad with grilled chicken
Dinner: Baked lemon herb chicken with roasted Brussels sprouts
Dessert: Mango slices

Day 16:

Breakfast: Avocado toast on whole-grain bread
Lunch: Lentil stew with whole-grain crackers
Dinner: Quinoa-stuffed bell peppers
Dessert: Frozen yogurt bark with berries

Day 17:

Breakfast: Chia seed pudding with sliced peaches

Lunch: Greek salad with grilled shrimp

Dinner: Baked herb-crusted cod with steamed asparagus

Dessert: Sliced watermelon

Day 18:

Breakfast: Scrambled eggs with diced tomatoes and herbs

Lunch: Quinoa salad with mixed vegetables and vinaigrette

Dinner: Baked lemon herb salmon with garlic mashed cauliflower

Dessert: Frozen grapes

Day 19:

Breakfast: Cottage cheese with pineapple and almonds

Lunch: Chicken and vegetable broth with whole-grain bread

Dinner: Grilled tofu with stir-fried vegetables and brown rice

Dessert: Baked apple slices with cinnamon

Day 20:

Breakfast: Greek yogurt parfait with berries and granola

Lunch: Bean salad with bell peppers and herbs

Dinner: Turkey stir-fry with quinoa

Dessert: Sliced strawberries with a dollop of whipped cream (in moderation)

Day 21:

Breakfast: Whole-grain toast with almond butter and sliced banana

Lunch: Hummus with veggie sticks and whole-grain crackers

Dinner: Eggplant parmesan (baked) with a side salad

Dessert: Mango sorbet

Day 22:

Breakfast: Spinach and feta omelet

Lunch: Cucumber and tomato salad with grilled chicken

Dinner: Roasted Brussels sprouts with baked lemon herb chicken

Dessert: Mixed fruit salad

Day 23:

Breakfast: Protein smoothie with kale, banana, and almond milk

Lunch: Tuna salad sandwich on whole-grain bread

Dinner: Baked herb-crusted tofu with quinoa and steamed broccoli

Dessert: Sliced pear with a sprinkle of cinnamon

Day 24:

Breakfast: Cottage cheese pancakes with fresh berries

Lunch: Greek salad with grilled shrimp

Dinner: Turkey chili with kidney beans and brown rice

Dessert: Baked apple slices with a touch of honey

Day 25:

Breakfast: Breakfast burrito with scrambled eggs, black beans, and salsa

Lunch: Caprese salad with grilled chicken

Dinner: Baked lemon herb salmon with roasted vegetables

Dessert: Greek yogurt with mixed fruits

Day 26:

Breakfast: Spinach and mushroom frittata

Lunch: Lentil soup with whole-grain crackers

Dinner: Stir-fried tofu with mixed vegetables and brown rice

Dessert: Banana "nice cream" made with frozen bananas

Day 27:

Breakfast: Overnight oats with chia seeds and mixed berries

Lunch: Mixed bean salad with bell peppers and vinaigrette

Dinner: Grilled swordfish with quinoa pilaf and roasted asparagus

Dessert: Watermelon slices

Day 28:

Breakfast: Breakfast quinoa with cinnamon and raisins
Lunch: Chicken Caesar salad with a light dressing
Dinner: Baked turkey meatballs with zucchini noodles
Dessert: Melon skewers

Day 29:

Breakfast: Smoothie bowl with spinach, banana, and almond milk topped with nuts and seeds
Lunch: Vegetable stir-fry with tofu
Dinner: Chicken and vegetable broth with whole-grain bread
Dessert: Mixed fruit salad with a drizzle of honey

Day 30:

Breakfast: Avocado toast on whole-grain bread

Lunch: Lentil stew with whole-grain crackers

Dinner: Quinoa-stuffed bell peppers

Dessert: Frozen yogurt bark with berries

Bonus 3

List of Medications You Never Knew were Killing Your Kidneys

When your kidneys do not operate properly, prescription and over-the-counter drugs can accumulate in your blood and cause more damage to your kidneys or other parts of your body. That is why persons with chronic kidney disease (CKD) must learn which treatments are appropriate for them and which are not. What medications should you avoid if you have kidney disease?

If you have kidney illness, your doctor may advise you to avoid or adjust your use of certain over-the-counter and prescription medications. If you are taking any of these medications, we urge that you consult with your doctor. Inform your doctor about all of your current drugs. Do not discontinue any medicine without first consulting your doctor.

- **Nonsteroidal anti-inflammatory medicines (NSAIDs) are pain relievers:** These drugs impair blood flow to the kidneys and should be avoided. NSAIDs are also present in many drugs used to treat fevers, colds, coughs, and sleep disorders. To be sure, always read the active ingredient labels on NSAIDs.

- **PPIs are proton pump inhibitors:** These drugs are used to treat acid reflux and heartburn, and some research suggests that they may raise the risk of renal disease, osteoporosis, and other nutritional deficiencies. If you are on dialysis, you may be restricted from using these medications. Before taking PPIs or other acid-reducing medications, always consult with your doctor.

- **Reflux Medication:** Statins (cholesterol-lowering drugs), These drugs are frequently recommended to help decrease blood cholesterol levels. To protect your kidneys, your doctor may consider the need to change the dosage of these medications.

- **Antibiotics:** Because antibiotics, antiviral, and antifungal drugs might injure your kidneys, your doctor must be informed of your kidney function before administering these medications.

- **Diabetes Medications:** Diabetes is the most common cause of renal disease. Diabetes patients must keep their blood sugar levels under control, which may necessitate the use of medication. If you have diabetes and are diagnosed with kidney disease, your doctor may need to change the dosage of your medication.

- **Antacids:** Over-the-counter heartburn and upset stomach drugs can disrupt your body's electrolyte balance, which can be troublesome for persons with chronic kidney disease. Before self-medicating, consult your doctor.

- **Vitamins and herbal supplements:** Many herbal supplements contain minerals that can be harmful to people with renal disease, such as potassium or phosphorus. In general, if you have renal illness, you should avoid herbal and vitamin supplements.

- **Contrast Dyes:** Contrast dyes used in diagnostic examinations like MRIs, CT scans, or angiograms may raise your risk of kidney issues or acute kidney injury (AKI). If you're scheduled for one of these tests, speak with the doctor who ordered it or your radiologist. Inform all healthcare providers involved in your care about your glomerular filtration rate (GFR) and CKD.

Dear Valued Reader,

Thank you for choosing our cookbook from the sea of options available. Your decision to embrace heart-healthy, plant-based living with us means the world. We invite you to share your thoughts by dropping a polite review on the website. Your feedback fuels our journey, and we're sincerely appreciative. Let your words be the heartbeat of our shared commitment to well-being. We also humbly ask you to consider checking out and following our author central page; with this, you will be exposed to a wealth of other books by this author.

With gratitude,

DR. AGISA BEGAY

Bonus 4

Meal Tracker / Journal

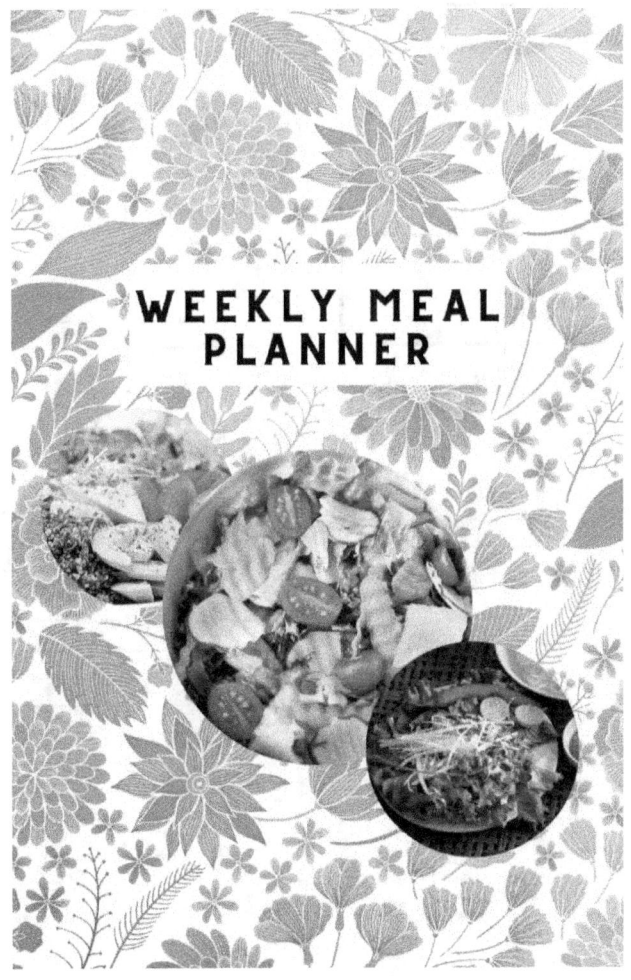

WEEK ____

s m t w t f s

Water ◆◆◆◆◆◆◆◆

Menu List :

Breakfast: _____

Lunch: _____

Dinner: _____

Dessert: _____

Snacks: _____

Priorities :

To do list :

Shopping List :

- ------------------------------
- ------------------------------
- ------------------------------
- ------------------------------
- ------------------------------
- ------------------------------
- ------------------------------
- ------------------------------
- ------------------------------
- ------------------------------
- ------------------------------
- ------------------------------
- ------------------------------
- ------------------------------

Notes and Tips :

_____
_____
_____
_____
_____
_____
_____
_____
_____
_____
_____

WEEK ____

s m t w t f s

Water ⬩⬩⬩⬩⬩⬩⬩⬩

Menu List :

Breakfast: _____

Lunch: _____

Dinner: _____

Dessert: _____

Snacks: _____

Priorities :

To do list :

Shopping List :

- ------------------------------
- ------------------------------
- ------------------------------
- ------------------------------
- ------------------------------
- ------------------------------
- ------------------------------
- ------------------------------
- ------------------------------
- ------------------------------
- ------------------------------
- ------------------------------
- ------------------------------
- ------------------------------

Notes and Tips :

WEEK ____

s m t w t f s

Water 🜄🜄🜄🜄🜄🜄🜄🜄

Menu List :

Breakfast:_____

Lunch:_____

Dinner:_____

Dessert:_____

Snacks:_____

Priorities :

To do list :

Shopping List :

- _____
- _____
- _____
- _____
- _____
- _____
- _____
- _____
- _____
- _____
- _____
- _____
- _____
- _____

Notes and Tips :

WEEK ____

s	m	t	w	t	f	s
●	●	●	●	●	●	●

Water ●●●●●●●

Menu List :

Breakfast: _____

Lunch: _____

Dinner: _____

Dessert: _____

Snacks: _____

Priorities :

To do list :

- -
- -
- -
- -
- -

Shopping List :

- ---------------------------------
- ---------------------------------
- ---------------------------------
- ---------------------------------
- ---------------------------------
- ---------------------------------
- ---------------------------------
- ---------------------------------
- ---------------------------------
- ---------------------------------
- ---------------------------------
- ---------------------------------
- ---------------------------------
- ---------------------------------

Notes and Tips :

WEEK _____

s m t w t f s

Water 🌢🌢🌢🌢🌢🌢🌢🌢

Menu List :

Breakfast: _____

Lunch: _____

Dinner: _____

Dessert: _____

Snacks: _____

Priorities :

To do list :

Shopping List :

- -------------------------------
- -------------------------------
- -------------------------------
- -------------------------------
- -------------------------------
- -------------------------------
- -------------------------------
- -------------------------------
- -------------------------------
- -------------------------------
- -------------------------------
- -------------------------------
- -------------------------------
- -------------------------------
- -------------------------------

Notes and Tips :

WEEK _____

s m t w t f s

Water ⬤⬤⬤⬤⬤⬤⬤

Menu List :

Breakfast: _____

Lunch: _____

Dinner: _____

Dessert: _____

Snacks: _____

Priorities :

To do list :

Shopping List :

- _____
- _____
- _____
- _____
- _____
- _____
- _____
- _____
- _____
- _____
- _____
- _____
- _____
- _____

Notes and Tips :

WEEK ____

s m t w t f s

Water

Menu List :

Breakfast: _____

Lunch: _____

Dinner: _____

Dessert: _____

Snacks: _____

Priorities :

To do list :

Shopping List :

- ----------------------------
- ----------------------------
- ----------------------------
- ----------------------------
- ----------------------------
- ----------------------------
- ----------------------------
- ----------------------------
- ----------------------------
- ----------------------------
- ----------------------------
- ----------------------------
- ----------------------------
- ----------------------------
- ----------------------------

Notes and Tips :

WEEK ____

s m t w t f s

Water 🌢🌢🌢🌢🌢🌢🌢🌢

Menu List :

Breakfast: _____

Lunch: _____

Dinner: _____

Dessert: _____

Snacks: _____

Priorities :

To do list :

Shopping List :

- --
- --
- --
- --
- --
- --
- --
- --
- --
- --
- --
- --
- --

Notes and Tips :

WEEK ____

s m t w t f s

Water

Menu List :

Breakfast: _____

Lunch: _____

Dinner: _____

Dessert: _____

Snacks: _____

Priorities :

To do list :

Shopping List :

- ----------------------------
- ----------------------------
- ----------------------------
- ----------------------------
- ----------------------------
- ----------------------------
- ----------------------------
- ----------------------------
- ----------------------------
- ----------------------------
- ----------------------------
- ----------------------------
- ----------------------------
- ----------------------------
- ----------------------------

Notes and Tips :

WEEK ____

s m t w t f s

Water

Menu List :

Breakfast: _____
Lunch: _____
Dinner: _____
Dessert: _____
Snacks: _____

Priorities :

To do list :

Shopping List :

- ----------------------------------
- ----------------------------------
- ----------------------------------
- ----------------------------------
- ----------------------------------
- ----------------------------------
- ----------------------------------
- ----------------------------------
- ----------------------------------
- ----------------------------------
- ----------------------------------
- ----------------------------------
- ----------------------------------
- ----------------------------------
- ----------------------------------

Notes and Tips :

Conclusion

Concluding this book, we will dedicate the following pages to do a recap of what we have discussed throughout this book.

Kidneys are vital organs located on either side of the spine, responsible for filtering blood and producing urine. They regulate the body's salt, potassium, and acid content and produce hormones. Chronic kidney disease, characterized by renal anomalies for three months or more, can be caused by diabetes, high blood pressure, glomerulonephritis, polycystic kidney disease, kidney stones, urinary tract infections, congenital disorders, and toxic substances. Symptoms include high blood pressure, urine containing blood and/or protein, higher creatinine and blood urea nitrogen levels, a GFR less than 60, frequent urination, puffiness around the eyes, and swelling in the hands and feet. Early detection and treatment are crucial to prevent kidney disease from advancing to kidney failure.

Chronic kidney disease (CKD) is a serious health issue that requires early detection and treatment. Risk factors include diabetes, high blood pressure, cardiovascular illness, kidney infections, long-term medication use, and autoimmune disorders. People with certain disorders, such as being older, having a family history of renal illness, or being of African or South Asian descent, are more likely to develop kidney disease. Diabetes is the leading cause of kidney disease in the US, affecting 6% of the population. High blood pressure affects one in every four Americans and is the second largest cause of renal disease. Controlling blood pressure can be achieved through lifestyle changes and regular exercise. A low glycemic diet can improve blood sugar control, weight loss, and potentially benefit those with a fatty liver.

The glycemic index (GI) is a dietary metric that measures the impact of carbohydrates on blood sugar levels. It is classified into low, medium, or high based on how quickly they elevate blood sugar levels. Eating low GI foods can reduce blood sugar spikes, while high GI foods can cause significant blood sugar rise. Glycemic load, an alternative metric, considers digestion rate and portion size. Eating low GI foods can help regulate blood sugar levels and aid in food pairings.

Kidney repair is crucial for maintaining a healthy lifestyle, especially for those with chronic renal disease. Healthful foods like apples, blueberries, fish, kale, spinach, and sweet potatoes can help prevent kidney damage. A kidney-friendly diet can be beneficial for those with diabetes and kidney disease, combining fruits, vegetables, protein sources, carbohydrates, and fluids. Dialysis patients may experience increased blood sugar levels due to high-sugar fluids. To avoid kidney disease, limit daily salt intake, use spices or herbs, and focus on fresh, home-cooked meals. Avoid potassium-rich foods, protein, phosphorus, calcium, and fluids, especially for early-stage renal disease patients. A recent study found a direct correlation between the amount of ultra-processed foods (UPFs) consumed and the risk of chronic kidney disease.

Inflammation is the body's natural defense against harmful substances, and an imbalanced diet, including processed foods like red meat, refined grains, snacks, sugary beverages, and fried foods, can lead to higher inflammation levels. These foods contain added sugars, saturated fats, and trans fats, and are often paired with alcohol. A balanced omega-6 to omega-3 fatty acid ratio is essential for preventing cardiovascular disease and cancer. Consuming antioxidant-rich foods is recommended for an anti-inflammatory diet. To reduce inflammation, restrict inflammation-causing meals and adopt a healthier, natural diet.

This book offers a variety of kidney-friendly food options, including soups, stews, appetizers, and snacks. It focuses on quick and easy dishes that maximize kidney function and prevent surgery. The recipes include vegetable quinoa soup, lentil stew, chicken and vegetable broth, and mestrone soup. Other options include hummus with vegetables, avocado with tortilla chips, rice cake with cottage cheese, baked lemon herb chicken, grilled salmon, turkey stir-fry, and eggplant parmesan.

The book offers a guide to meal planning for people with chronic kidney disease (CKD), emphasizing understanding kidney health requirements, monitoring nutrients, and creating a balanced diet plan. It emphasizes limiting sodium, phosphorous intake, and consuming low-potassium foods. Nutrition labels should be read for kidney-friendly choices, and portion sizes should be calculated. Eating kidney-friendly meals throughout the day, including high-protein breakfasts, balanced lunches, and desserts with fresh fruits and grains, is crucial for overall health.

Chronic kidney disease patients should avoid certain medications like NSAIDs, PPIs, statins, antibiotics, diabetes treatments, and herbal supplements, as they can impair kidney function and increase the risk of renal disease, osteoporosis, and nutritional deficiencies. Doctors should prescribe antibiotics, antiviral, and antifungal drugs based on kidney function.

Kidney disease is never a death sentence, there have been countless survivors of this illness around the world. With the proper knowledge, nutritional adjustment and lifestyle management, kidney disease will be a thing of the past. I advise you make the best of dietary choices, healing truly exist in a plate!

Dear Valued Reader,

Thank you for choosing our cookbook from the sea of options available. Your decision to embrace heart-healthy, plant-based living with us means the world. We invite you to share your thoughts by dropping a polite review on the website. Your feedback fuels our journey, and we're sincerely appreciative. Let your words be the heartbeat of our shared commitment to well-being. We also humbly ask you to consider checking out and following our author central page; with this, you will be exposed to a wealth of other books by this author.

With gratitude,

DR. AGISA BEGAY

Acknowledgement

Picture Links

https://images.pexels.com/photos/9705830/pexels-photo-9705830.jpeg?auto=compress&cs=tinysrgb&w=600&lazy=load

https://images.pexels.com/photos/9705821/pexels-photo-9705821.jpeg?auto=compress&cs=tinysrgb&w=600&lazy=load

https://www.freepik.com/free-photo/top-view-colorful-vegetables-lentil-bowl-colorful-vegetables-spices_13292494.htm

https://www.freepik.com/free-photo/top-view-cucumbers-with-broccoli_12418216.htm

www.ingramcontent.com/pod-product-compliance
Lightning Source LLC
Chambersburg PA
CBHW072154290526
45794CB00004B/1509